MW00365384

The Art of Life

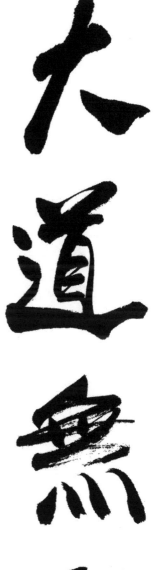

Simon Blow

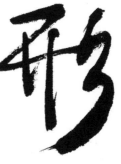

First published 2010
Second Edition 2013
Copyright © 2010 Simon Blow

National Library of Australia
Cataloguing-in-Publication data:

Simon Blow

The Art of Life

ISBN: 978-0-9750480-9-2

Published by:
The Genuine Wisdom Centre
PO Box 446
Summer Hill NSW 2130
Australia
(www.genuinewisdomcentre.com)

Editing:
Essence Writing (www.essencewriting.com.au)

Cover design and layout:
Determind Design (www.determind.com.au)

Diagrams:
Avril Carruthers and John Bennetts

Disclaimer
The intention of this book is to present information and practices that have been used throughout China for many years. The information offered is according to the author's best knowledge and is to be used by the reader at his or her own discretion and liability. Readers should obtain professional advice where appropriate regarding their health and health practices. The author disclaims all responsibility and liability to any person, arising directly or indirectly from taking or not taking action based upon the information in this publication.

This book is dedicated to

… all those who are facing challenges in their life

Contents

Acknowledgements

There are many people I would like to thank for helping me to compile and develop this book.

Since I started teaching full-time in 1992, I have taught 18 to 22 classes per week – the best way to learn something is to teach it, as the old saying goes. This is especially relevant when working with the universal life force Qi energy, as it is important to be in front of people to share this energy. Qigong Master Jack Lim told me that when you are teaching a class, think of it as being with a group of friends and sharing. Thank you for this advice, Jack.

I would like to thank all those friends who have attended my classes and workshops over the years. I get many ideas and positive feedback from the students and people I meet, and from those who have generously shared their own experiences. I am not sure if we have original ideas or if, when the heart opens and the Qi flows, we are simply all one. Again, thank you.

I would like to thank Lynn Guilhaus for proofreading, editing, researching and additional writing and for bringing this project to life. Thanks to John Kooyman for the original photos of the Standing Ba Duan Jin and Taiji Qigong Shibashi, and to Avril Carruthers for the wonderful illustrations. They are all works of art. Thank you to John Bennetts for the original photos and adaptations to drawings for the Qigong warm-up and Master Zhang Cheng Cheng and Master Liu Changlin for the Chinese writing. Thank you to Adriene Hurst for additional editing, Ivan Finnegan for original cover design and Mamun Khan from Determind Design for the layout and design of the book and my friends at Bashundhara Printing.

We refer to Qigong as an art form. It is a process of refining our internal energy to harmonise with the external energy or environment. It is our own observation of our relationship with everything around us. We are influenced by everything around us, we are one with everything.

I have had the fortunate opportunity to meet many great masters, professors and doctors, but mainly, just great people who are committed to contributing to the development of the human race. Thank you.

Foreword

I first met Simon Blow in 1983 in a personal development and meditation class. A few years later, some of us in that meditation class shared a house with Simon and I got to know him as a gentle person with a quiet sense of his own individuality. Unlike many others in their twenties, Simon was rarely swayed by fads and fashions or by what others thought important. He seemed to follow his own inner vision with calm certainty. However, it was evident that he was also open-minded about many different avenues of self-development and spiritual awareness and was searching for answers.

We lost touch for a few years while I began my psychotherapy practice and continued my studies in meditation with the Clairvision School in Sydney. In the early nineties I felt I needed to extend my meditation practice with an exploration into Tai Chi. I tried a couple of different teachers but was unimpressed by the experience until I happened to walk into a class taught by my old friend Simon. This wasn't the only surprise. The class itself and the sense of Simon's presence were extraordinary. I felt my energy revive and flow in a peaceful harmony. I knew I would have a long association with this gentle energy form.

I was familiar with martial arts. In the sixties I had studied judo as a child and in the seventies enthusiastically took it up again along with two other Japanese martial arts – Karate and Ju-Jitsu. I learnt Zen Buddhist meditation with it. I learnt about energy and in particular, about Ki – known in Chinese as Chi or Qi. It fascinated me that using Ki, a small person such as myself could overpower a much stronger, larger one, using the weight and momentum of the opponent. When pushed, I learnt to pull. When pulled, I learnt to push. In another Japanese form, Aikido, I learnt about the power of circularity of momentum in throwing an opponent. I was very much into the Warrior archetype. I loved fighting, pitting force against force, seeking the weakness in my opponent. Overcoming obstacles, being unstoppable and seeking challenges in all areas of my life were all part of it – but they were also somewhat of a diversion and more inner work was needed in my life to balance the extreme physicality of these martial arts. I plunged more deeply into meditation. Work and family commitments then took over and I let go of the martial arts for a period. Ten years later, when I met Simon again in his Tai Chi class, my body had slowed down enough for the fighting spirit of the Warrior to be replaced by something gentler and wiser. I realised Simon was embodying the next stage of my journey. He became my teacher. At the same time I was retracing the history of unarmed martial arts itself, back to the practices of Shaolin warrior monks in China around the 7th century CE.

Because Tai Chi is a soft form and more about health than combat, it is not an obvious choice for a person who likes fighting and force-against-force. In fact, when I had tried it once in my mid-twenties I found it incomprehensible. Who wanted to move so slowly? I just didn't get it. I had to slow down altogether for it to make sense to me. I needed a certain maturity. By then, I knew from my martial arts training that intention can command the direction of Ki within the body. After all, with intention, concentration between the eyebrows and Ki, I could break a piece of solid pine planking with my hand or foot. When it came to Tai Chi, I found the principle was the same, though there was no force at all. Intention allowed Qi to flow from my core, my lower Dan Tian, through my entire body, or from my feet to the crown of my head or my fingertips. The vibrational flow was inherently healing. I could feel it as it moved powerfully along the meridians and through the organs. It balanced me. I felt calm and energised. It increased the awareness I had already developed in my meditation practices. It deepened my healing practice with clients. Before long, I also became an instructor of Tai Chi, for a time teaching alongside Simon and then branching into my own classes.

Simon's studies expanded into Qigong, a more profound form of intentional inner energy flow that originated 5,000 years ago in ancient Traditional Chinese Medicine, and that, he has now naturally passed on to his students. It is the main subject of this book. For many years, in addition to my own daily practice, Simon and I met weekly for Qigong practice under the trees in the park, through all the seasons of the year, much as people in China do daily. We'd then go back to my meditation room to meditate for an hour. It was an enriching process in both our lives.

I am privileged to write the foreword to this, Simon's first book, and delighted to have provided the illustrations. Through the more than quarter-century that I have known him, I've been constantly impressed with his calm persistence and single-mindedness. Living what he teaches, Simon's achievements mirror the wisdom of the Dao De Jing of Lao-Tzu in its description of water.

The highest good is like water,
Water nourishes the Ten Thousand Things
Without striving with them.
VIII

From his early battle to overcome devastating injuries due to a car accident as a teenager, to the ongoing pursuit of his vision to help others overcome their own challenges, Master Simon Blow embodies the true archetypes of Peaceful Warrior and Teacher. If you are lucky enough to be in one of his classes, you will have experienced the calm that emanates from him. If you have one of his beautifully produced Qigong DVDs, in which black swans and ducks peacefully forage a few feet away from Simon under the trees, you'll be able to feel it too. In the practice of this healing art, you will discover your own serenity and balance of body and spirit. May this book enrich your life.

Avril Carruthers BA M.Couns.
Sydney, November 2009.

About the Author: Simon Blow

A near-fatal accident at the age of nineteen lead Simon to investigate various methods of healing and rejuvenation, a path he has been following ever since. Simon is a Sydney-based (Australia) master teacher (Laoshi) of the ancient Chinese art of longevity and has been leading regular classes for beginning and continuing students since 1990.

Having travelled the world to learn and explore this ancient art, Simon has received extensive training and certification from many respected sources: Traditional Chinese Medical Hospitals and Daoist Monasteries in China, Buddhist Monasteries in Australia, and Hindu Ashrams in India. He has been given authority to share these techniques through his teachings and publications.

Simon received World Health Organisation Certification in Medical Qigong clinical practice from the Xiyuan Hospital in Beijing and is a Standing Council Member of the World Academic Society of Medical Qigong in Beijing. He has also been initiated into Dragon Gate Daoism and given the name of Xin Si, meaning Genuine Wisdom.

His dedication, compassion and wisdom also make Simon a sought-after keynote speaker and workshop facilitator. By demand he has created a series of Book/DVD sets and guided meditation CDs. He also helps produce CDs for the Sunnatram Forest Monastery, the YWCA Encore program and a series of Meditation CDs for children and teenagers.

China holds a special place in Simon's heart. He has had the great fortune to travel to China on many occasions to study Qigong, attend international conferences, tour the sacred mountains and experience the rich culture of the Chinese people. Since 1999 he has been leading unique study tours to China so he could take people to the source and give them the opportunity to experience first-hand this ancient healing practice.

Romanisation of Chinese words

The Genuine Wisdom Centre uses the Pinyin romanisation system of Chinese to English. Pinyin is a name for the system used to transliterate Chinese words into the Roman alphabet. The use of Pinyin was first adopted in the 1950s by the Chinese government, and it became official in 1979 when it was endorsed by the People's Republic of China.

Pinyin is now standard in the People's Republic of China and in several world organisations, including the United Nations. Pinyin replaces the Wade-Giles and Yale systems.

Some common conversions:

Pinyin	Also spelled as	Pronunciation
Qi	Chi	Chee
Qigong	Chi Kung	Chee Kung
Taiji	Tai Chi	Tai Jee
Taijiquan	Tai Chi Chuan	Tai Jee Chuen
Gongfu	Kung Fu	Gong Foo
Dao	Tao	Dao
Daoism	Taoism	Daoism
Dao De Jing	Tao Teh Ching	Dao Teh Ching

How to use this book

Traditionally we follow the teacher/master and this balances our energy. The book gives detailed instructions on how to perform the movements and provides additional theory and history to complement the practises. To view videos showing the shape of the movements please visit our YouTube channel
www.yoututbe.com/simonblowqigong

It's important to learn from an experienced qualified teacher and to practise regularly to master the movements yourself. Attending regular classes provides consistent practice and refinement and the energy of the group nurtures and supports everyone. It's important not to stray too far from the flock.

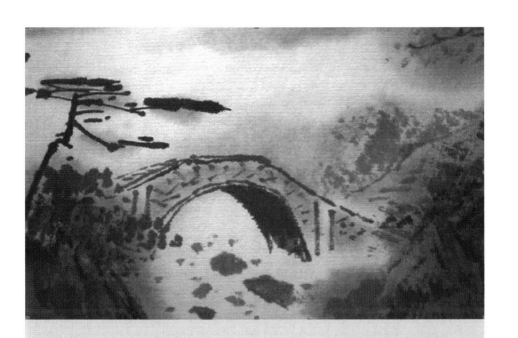

Chapter 1

Introduction

The Art of Life

Introduction

Qigong (Chi Kung), and the understanding of Qi (Chi), is one of the great treasures of Chinese culture. It has emerged over thousands of years from constant research, development and practice. From ancient times to the modern world, we as human beings are on a continuous journey of self-enquiry to discover our true identity and purpose in life.

Qigong originated in China as a way of cultivating spiritual, physical and emotional health. Similarly, other cultures had holistic approaches to connect and harmonise with their local environment and their known universe. When we lose this connection it causes problems and we are not able to enjoy the experience of life as much as we could.

> *"When you are proud of your achievement it is time to stop.*
> *If you sharpen and strengthen your mind by taking advantage of people, your enjoyment will not last long.*
> *One who accumulates valuable things will not be able to maintain them without becoming a slave to them.*
> *Becoming rich and noble with pride is to invite trouble for oneself.*
> *After accomplishing one's goal it is time to retreat.*
> *This is the way of Heaven."*
>
> Lao Tzu, Dao De Jing. Chapter Nine

Its origins trace back to the Tangyao period of 4,000-5,000 years ago. It was clearly outlined in the book Huangdi Neijing or The Yellow Emperor's Internal Canon of Chinese Medicine, which in 2,500 BC described the basic theory of Traditional Chinese Medicine and is still used today.

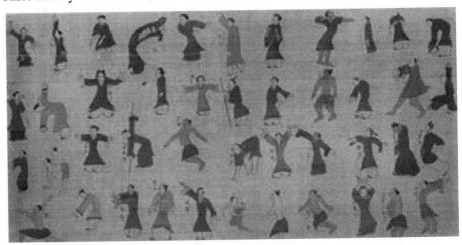

Daoyin Diagrams

Medical books published from the Han Dynasty 200 BC show detailed theory and clinical practice of Qigong techniques for treating disease and improving health. Silk scrolls known as the Daoyin Diagrams, unearthed in 1972 at an archaeological dig in Changsha, China, show detailed illustrations of medical Qigong exercises and have been dated to 168 BC.

Qigong is a relatively new term to describe all the Chinese energy or Qi techniques. Qi or Chi is a term meaning 'life force energy' that flows through the energy channels or meridians in the body and connects with the energy of the universe. Gong or Gung translates as work, mastery or skill – literally, a way of working with the energy of life. There are three main categories of Qigong: Martial, Medical and Spiritual. The Qigong methods described in this book relate to medical/healing and spiritual Qigong.

The art of Qigong consists primarily of meditation, relaxation, physical movement, mind-body integration and breathing exercises. There are thousands of different styles and systems, either done standing, moving, walking, sitting or lying. Tai Chi is one popular style.

For thousands of years, millions of people have benefited from Qigong practice. From ancient to modern times, Qigong self-healing exercises have been used to help improve people's quality of life. In Traditional Chinese Medicine, good health is a result of a free-flowing, well-balanced energy system. Ailments, both physical and emotional, occur when the flow of Qi is blocked or impeded, causing imbalance and dysfunction in the body's energy system. With regular practice, Qigong helps to cleanse the body of toxins, restore energy, reduce stress and anxiety, and help individuals maintain a healthy and active life.

Qi – the essence of life

Qi (pronounced Chi) is the foundation of Taoist thinking and Traditional Chinese Medicine (TCM) and is described by Taoist Master Hua-Ching Ni in his book, *Tao – the Subtle Universal Law and the Integral Way of Life*:

"Chi is the vital universal energy that composes, permeates and moves everything that exists. Chi may be defined as the ultimate cause and, at the same time, the ultimate effect of all activity. Chi is the ultimate essence of the universe as well as the law of all movement. When Chi conglomerates, it is called matter. When Chi is diffuse, it is called space. When Chi animates form it is called life. When Chi separates

*and withdraws, it is called death. When Chi flows, there is health.
When Chi is blocked, there is sickness and disease. Chi embraces,
circulates through and sustains all things. The planets depend on
Chi to regulate their atmosphere, light, weather and the seasons.*

*"So, it is Chi or vital energy that activates and maintains all life. Chi
animates all the processes of the body: the digestion and assimilation
of the food we eat, the inhalation and exhalation of air by the lungs,
the circulation of the blood, the dissemination of fluids throughout
the body and, finally, the excretion of waste products."*

This flow of energy or Qi in our body is directly related to our posture
and body movements, breath and mental condition. When the mind, body
and breath are in harmony, our Qi will also be in harmony. It will flow
naturally through the energy channels or meridians of the body, allowing
us to connect with the energy of the universe.

When we practise Qigong, it's important not to try too hard. Most forms
of Qigong involve gentle movements, balanced with rhythmical, regulated
breathing, and in a calm, focused and unhurried way. Take your time and
allow the movements and breath to develop. In the classic text called
Spring and Autumn Annals, the sage Confucius says:

*"Flowing water never stagnates, and the hinges of an active door
never rust. This is due to movement. The same principle applies to
essence and energy. If the body does not move, essence does not flow.
When essence does not flow, energy stagnates."*

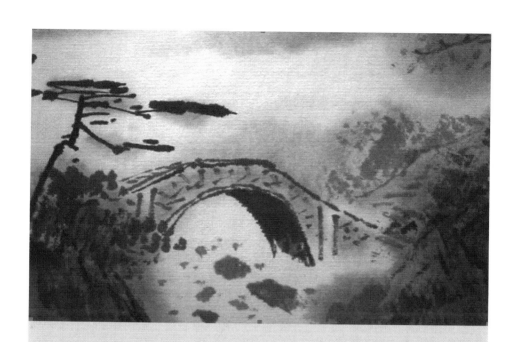

Chapter 2

The Benefits of Qigong

The Art of Life

The Benefits of Qigong

Why practice Qigong?

The emphasis on the spiritual life, rather than the material life, is one of the major differences between eastern and western cultures. For example, western medicine emphasises the physical body and the treatment of ailments through medication. Eastern medicine tends to treat the person's spiritual and mental health and has a greater focus on prevention, quality of life and longevity.

Many people believe that by exercising hard they will achieve an externally strong body and will be healthier and happier. But to have good health it is necessary to have a healthy body, healthy mind and balanced Qi circulation. According to Chinese medicine, many illnesses are caused by imbalances in the mind. For example, worry and nervousness can upset the stomach. Fear can affect the functioning of the kidneys and bladder. The internal energy (Qi) is closely related to the mind. To be truly healthy, one must have both a healthy physical body and a calm and healthy mind.

> *"After 15 years of training at the gym I was suffering from a bad shoulder which kept me away from training. After just a few weeks of practising Qigong my shoulder pain decreased. I also find it relaxing and calming and intend to make Qigong a life-time practice."* Julie Meehan

Too much of something is excessive Yang and too little is excessive Yin. When the body is too Yang or too Yin, the internal organs will tend to weaken and degenerate more rapidly. When we get older, body tissue begins to degenerate and this causes Qi to stagnate in the Qi channels. Movement is a manifestation of Yang activity, and stillness reflects the calmness of Yin. In today's hectic world, overactivity causes Fire to flare up and uses one's reserves of essence and energy, while the stillness of meditation cools the Fire, calms the system, and conserves vital resources.

For health improvement and maintenance, the Qigong participant does not have to be an expert. Anyone can learn to practise Qigong. The objective of the exercises is to strengthen the Qi in the body and remove obstructions to Qi flow that may have developed due to injury, diet, disease, emotional states, or other factors.

"I have been practising Qigong for about five years and practise six days per week. It constantly amazes me how something that appears so simple can give me such a feeling of wellbeing and inner harmony." Neville Webb

Of all the energy medical practices, Qigong has been subjected to the most extensive research. In China, Medical Qigong is now practiced in clinics and some hospitals that integrate Traditional Chinese Medicine (TCM) and conventional Western medicine. In Western hospitals Qigong is among several complementary practices used including therapeutic touch and mindful meditation.

"Qi is the energy of life.
It's cultivated through work expressed as creativity,
shared through humanity, enabling us to merge with the universe,
returning to nothingness" Simon Blow

Clinical research demonstrates the multifaceted effects of Qigong

In the early 1980s Chinese scientists initiated research on the health and healing claims of Qigong. Of the hundreds of research studies that were performed, few were published because suitable journals were unavailable. However, about 1,400 reports were published as abstracts in the proceedings of conferences. English abstracts of these reports as well as those from scientific journals are collected in the Qigong and Energy Database that presently contains more than 5,000 abstracts of Qigong studies and is available from the Qigong Institute (Sancier KM 2000). **www.qigonginstitute.org**

One of the prime benefits of Qigong is stress reduction, and a main ingredient of practice is intention (i.e., Yi). Intention uses the mind to guide the Qi. While Qi itself has not been measured, different physiological measurements have sought information about the effects of Qigong on the brain and emotions. These include measurements by high-resolution electroencephalography (EEG), functional MRI (fMRI), neurometer measurements, and applied kinesiology.

Neuroimaging methods were used to study regional brain functions, emotions and disorders of emotions. Differences were found on the effects on the brain during meditation by Qigong and by Zen meditation. (Kawano K 1996). The effects of emitted Qi (waiqi) has also been extended to cell cultures, growth of plants, seed germination, and reduction of tumor size in animals (Sancier KM 1991).

Spiritual healing, which involves the mind, has been the subject of two volumes by Benor (Benor DJ 2001; Benor DJ 2002). His discussions also include scientific studies describing the beneficial effects of prayer on subjects' health.

The work of Richard Davidson and Paul Ekman, researchers of the Mind and Life Institute, may go a long way to illustrate the role of intention alone on the brain and body (Davidson JD 1999). In current studies underway at the University of California, San Francisco Medical School and University of Wisconsin, they are observing the electrical mechanisms in the brains of highly trained Buddhist lamas during various states of focused intention. Using functional MRI, high-resolution EEG and state-of-the art reflex monitoring, their early results illustrate that electrical activity and blood flow in the brain can be directed by conscious intention.

Through systematic and repeated practice of intention, well-practiced lamas have succeeded in training the brain to direct electrical activity away from areas associated with the biochemistry of stress, tension and disturbing emotional or physical states (i.e., the amygdala and right prefrontal cortex) and increase activity in the area associated with the biochemistry of healthful emotional and physical states (i.e., the left prefrontal cortex). Moreover, they have observed that the state of conscious intention on compassion engages a state of relaxation and wellbeing which surpasses even that achieved during a state of rest. The early results of this research suggests that parts of the brain, thought previously to be fixed in function, such as the stress reflexes of the reptilian brain, may in fact be plastic in nature, able to be changed, shaped and developed through ongoing practice of conscious intention.(Lama Dalai 2003).

Adapted from: Multifaceted Health Benefits of Medical Qigong, *J. Alt Compl Med.* 2004; 10(1):163-166, by Kenneth M. Sancier, Ph.D. & Devatara Holman MS, MA, Lac.

Survey of benefits of Qigong practice with a drug rehabilitation population
(Extract)

By Simon Blow, presented at the World Medical Qigong Conference, Beijing 2004.

Overview: The problem of addiction is a huge one causing breakdown of family and community structure, disruption to work, crime and civil disorder. Research suggests the causes lie in childhood abuse, parental alcoholism and neglect, resulting in a downward spiral of low self-esteem, powerlessness, violence and self-harm. Addicts are therefore often individuals in a state of extreme imbalance – physically, mentally, spiritually and emotionally. When they decide to address their substance abuse, changing themselves, their attitudes and habits, it is a struggle.

The ancient practice of Qigong has long been known in China and increasingly in the west as a means of increasing health and wellbeing. Over the past twelve years Qigong Master Simon Blow has been leading classes in Ba Duan Jin Standing Form Qigong in several drug rehabilitation groups in Sydney, Australia. The practice of Qigong as taught by Simon Blow utilises the elements of self-healing and balance of the internal energy with the external environment. The results suggest that the practice of Qigong gives beneficial aid to recovering addicts in gaining relaxation skills, body awareness and confidence as well as lessening frustration and regaining balance of body and mind.

The survey: A survey was taken continuously over six months from June to December 2003 after each 45-minute class of Qigong, held twice weekly, in a residential, drug rehabilitation group. We Help Ourselves (WHOS), is a three-month drug-free therapeutic program that incorporates the fostering of personal growth and life skills with a view to participants returning to the community. The context of these Qigong classes is therefore a therapeutic one of groupwork, counselling, support and education, stress management and relapse prevention.

Two groups of males and females were surveyed over two consecutive three-month periods with the intention of a qualitative assessment based on subjective evaluation on whether their on-going Qigong practice was helping in their recovery.

Results: Of a total of 634 surveys over this period, 89% found an overall benefit. Specific qualities were measured: 85% said they felt stronger physically; 86% said they were able to accept others more and 87% felt that their self-acceptance had increased; 88% felt the practice of Qigong enabled them to concentrate better and felt more confident and better able to control anxiety; 88% felt they were deepening spiritually; 89% felt stronger emotionally and less frustrated; 90% felt Qigong practice was an important routine and that they were more aware of Qi; 92% felt Qigong was an important part of their recovery; 93% said they felt more peaceful since learning Qigong and that their future would be a better one; 95% felt Qigong helped them to be calm and relaxed.

Participant comments

- *I feel more centred on the days that we practise.*
- *I have slowed down a lot and my thoughts are not so chaotic.*
- *(After practice I feel) calm, peaceful and clear of mind. (I find it) amazing.*
- *I have struggled with substance abuse and when I came into a rehabilitation program that practised Qigong I was extremely reluctant in the beginning and negative about Qigong. I decided to give it a go with a positive outlook and now I enjoy it. I feel better after the session and also it is a good form of exercise which I enjoy.*
- *I am learning to relax on my own.*
- *Qigong has helped me to relax more on a daily basis and go more within myself to find inner happiness. It has helped give me a nice balance between body, mind and soul. Qigong has been a stepping stone for me to introduce more exercise and meditation into my daily program.*
- *I can concentrate more on the days we practise.*
- *I feel calmer. I like it when we throw the bad energy out. (It) feels good.*
- *A sense of peace, more balanced and (I have) a better understanding of myself.*
- *I feel that I can relax and get to sleep a lot easier. Also I know what my body is telling me. Thank you.*
- *I'm more willing to be embarrassed.*
- *(I've developed) more motor skills and (am) centred.*
- *I find the movements easier to do and become more relaxed and focused after our session.*

- *I find I have slowed down a bit.*
- *It makes me feel good about myself.*
- *I feel more peaceful about myself and also feel good and happy about life.*
- *(I am more) calm, peaceful and aware.*
- *(I am) stronger, more courageous, more serene, more calm.*
- *(I am) more willing to try. I felt more relaxed and warm. Not so embarrassed.*
- *I feel more connected to myself and my higher power.*
- *(After practice I feel) relaxed, yawning, hungry.*
- *When doing Qigong I can feel the hair on my upper body stand up. It is really relaxing. I find myself looking forward to the classes and talk to my peers about it. I find myself easy to be with the day I do it. I feel my body in a way I never have before.*
- *(I find it) good to stretch. I am learning patience (with Qigong). (It) keeps my mind open.*
- *(I am) more relaxed and it helps with my aches and pains.*
- *(I am) more self aware and more aware of my body. I have learned to recognise my feelings and be less stressed about them more often.*
- *I feel Qigong is balancing my two sides – female and male. I have noticed I have resistance to just letting go, my right side is more energetically activated. Now it is more balanced.*
- *(Qigong is) very good for my recovery, to calm myself down.*
- *I am able to feel my emotions a lot more.*
- *I am more aware of what is happening in my life.*

Conclusion: The first step to changing oneself is awareness. In helping these participants become more aware of themselves and their bodies, as well as in helping them relax and become less stressed about the emotions they are discovering, the practice of Qigong is demonstrably a method for helping people change. It is a significant aid to this rehabilitation program.

For more research on the Scientific Basis of Qigong and Energy Medicine visit **http://www.qigonginstitute.org/html/papers.php**

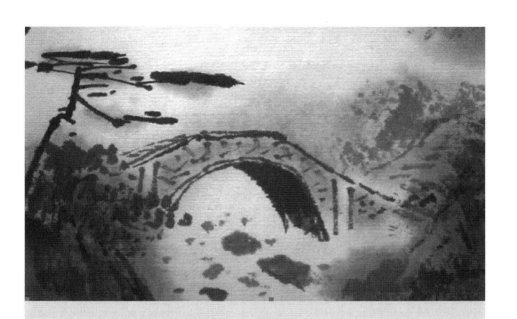

Chapter 3

Meditation and Health – the Research

The Art of Life

Meditation and Health – the Research

The three main principles of Qigong practice are the concentration of body movements, the breath and the mind. Qigong has both a dynamic (Yang) and stillness (Yin) component. Qigong can be referred to as a mindful or meditation practice.

The term *meditation* refers to a variety of techniques or practices intended to focus or control attention. Most meditative techniques are rooted in Eastern religious or spiritual traditions and have been used by many different cultures throughout the world for thousands of years. Today, many people use meditation outside of its traditional religious or cultural settings to improve their health and wellness.

Researchers have been collecting data on meditation for many years and countless studies have shown that meditation has not only a mental but a physiological effect on the body. Many of the findings show that, among other benefits, meditation can help reverse heart disease, reduce pain and enhance the body's immune system.

In one area of research, scientists are using sophisticated tools to determine possible changes in brain function. With the use of MRI technology, researchers at Harvard Medical School found that meditation affects parts of the brain that are in charge of the autonomic nervous system which governs the functions of our organs, muscles and body systems. Stress compromises these functions so it makes sense to harmonise these functions to help ward off stress-related conditions such as heart disease, digestive problems and infertility.

In a study published in the journal *Stroke*, a control group of 60 people with atherosclerosis, or hardening of the arteries, practised meditation for six to nine months. The meditators showed a decrease in the thickness of their artery walls, while the non-meditators actually showed an increase. The change for the meditation group could potentially decrease their risk of heart attack by 11% and the risk of stroke by 8-15%.

Another study, published in *Psychosomatic Medicine*, taught mindful meditation to a group of 90 cancer patients. After seven weeks, those who meditated reported that they were less depressed, anxious, angry and confused than the control group, which hadn't practised meditation. The meditators also had more energy and fewer heart and gastrointestinal problems than did the other group.

Researchers for a study published in the *Public Library of Science* shows that peaceful thoughts can influence our bodies, right down to the instructions we receive from our DNA. Researchers took blood samples from a group of 19 people who habitually meditated or prayed for years, and 19 others who never meditated. They found that the meditating group suppressed more than twice the number of stress-related genes – about 1,000 of them – than the non-meditating group.

The more these stress-related genes are expressed, the more the body will have a stress response, and over long periods of time these stress responses can increase inflammation, and worsen high blood pressure, pain syndromes and other conditions. According to leading researcher Dr Herbert Benson, an associate professor of medicine at Harvard Medical School, meditation breaks the train of everyday thought thereby reducing stressful thoughts and allowing the body to return to a healthy state.

Dr Dean Ornish, professor of medicine and founder of the Preventive Medicine Research Institute at the University of California at San Francisco, recently found a relationship between meditation and genes in prostate cancer. These preliminary findings suggest that meditation, when combined with better nutrition and moderate exercise, might favorably alter gene expression in prostate tissue.

Another small study published in *Menopause: The Journal of the North American Menopause Society*, showed that menopausal women who participated in a stress reduction program that included meditation experienced significant relief from hot flashes and improvements in their quality of life.

While western scientists are still exploring exactly how and why meditation works, we already know that it has both physiological and psychological benefits. Many therapists now consider it a valid complement to more traditional therapies and anything that helps fight stress is a welcome tool.

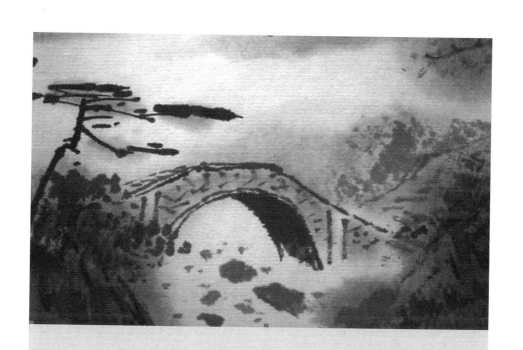

Chapter 4

The Art of Life

The Art of Life

The Art of Life

I meet many people who are on a healing journey and I hear countless stories of how tragic accidents or illnesses have become turning points, changing their lives.

My own healing story is not unusual or remarkable, but I made a decision to change and deliberately set out on a course that gave me an opportunity to grow.

I enjoyed a normal upbringing. My father was a country bank manager and our family moved around the NSW region of Australia. We had a middle-class lifestyle with regular family holidays and lots of love and support. In the late 1970s I followed my father into the bank as this offered a good, stable career path. I enjoyed being a country bank teller – an honest, trustworthy occupation at that time. People trusted bank tellers and would share stories about their lives. I was an active, athletic teenager, playing most sports. I was never the star player but always an enthusiastic member of the team. I was a normal kid discovering life.

But life was about to change!

It was Boxing Day, 1979 when my family was told to prepare for the worst as I lay in hospital in intensive care, attached to a life support system. They were told that, if I lived, the injuries I had sustained in a head-on collision meant I might never be able to lead a normal life. This accident marked the start of a new stage of my life and an awakening to a new reality.

I don't remember much about the first six weeks in hospital and I have no memory of the accident that put me there. I sustained fractures to both feet, both ankles and legs, and suffered a fractured arm, shoulder and collarbone, and severe head injuries. Only my right arm escaped injury from the high-speed impact. While the occupants of the other vehicle had received only minor injuries, I had borne the full brunt of the collision and would have to live with the consequences for the rest of my life.

I was admitted to a Catholic Hospital. In the chapel, the nuns kept praying that my life be spared. I nearly died on a few occasions that first week in intensive care. I was nineteen years old but had I been older, in my 40s, I would not have survived. My journey was about to start and it was going to be a long hard road to walk.

My left foot was severely injured and had to be wired back together. My right femur, or thigh bone, was shattered and set in traction. I was confined to bed with a heavy weight pulling the bones apart to allow them to heal. Because I wasn't responding emotionally, the doctors were worried that I may have a brain injury but CAT scans showed no abnormalities. It was as though the lights inside had dimmed and I wasn't there.

After nine weeks when I could be moved, I made my first clear decision to change. In order to be transported to another hospital closer to my family, I was taken out of traction and placed in a plaster cast from my foot to under my ribs to encase my badly injured right leg. It was a harrowing experience as nurses and physiotherapists held me to apply the plaster. When the doctor came later that day to inspect the job, he found the cast hadn't been made correctly and would have to be cut off and done again. The next day as they sawed off the hard plaster and applied the new cast, I grew frustrated and angry and suddenly realised the nature of the situation I was in. From that moment, I committed to getting better.

That decision, together with the 400km road ambulance trip and a new hospital and surroundings, 'woke' me up. The lights came on and have remained on ever since.

After three months, I remember quite clearly starting to walk again. Using a walking frame, I would very slowly and carefully walk around the ward. I was so excited that I was making progress. One of the nurses would lead me to other patients who were feeling down and depressed, encouraging me to tell my story. I could see the change in their eyes and the healing process taking place. Since that day I have been inspired to share all that I learn and know, to be able to receive more.

After the initial three months in hospital, I underwent four years of intensive physical rehabilitation but, after several structural operations, one of Australia's leading orthopaedic surgeons finally told me I must accept the fact that I would never again lead an active life.

There are many ways to heal. To clear pain physically and emotionally we need to start by accepting our condition and seeking the appropriate action to initiate the healing process in our self. My life was in the balance that first week in hospital, I nearly died from embolisms or clots that occurred from the multiple fractures that I sustained. When my condition stabilised I knew I was going to recover, but did not know to what level of recovery and what quality of life I would have. After a few months I remember looking around the orthopaedic ward and seeing all the other accident victims, some I would talk to and we would discuss our injuries and the circumstances that put us there. I could sense in some people that they had given up, but I was determined to get better and to continue with my life.

I was a good patient and what the doctors and physiotherapists told me to do I did, and then did more. I was told to accept my situation, to know my limitations and work with that. I haven't been able to run since the accident. I can run across the road if a car is approaching, but I can't play any type of running sport like tennis or basketball. Even long walks can aggravate unnecessary pain.

Over the next few years I tried to live a normal life. I worked in the international department of a large bank, enjoyed my job as a supervisor and team leader, and thrived by helping people and solving problems. I was trying to be normal but I realised I wasn't normal. I seemed to have a deeper understanding and insight and felt much older than my age. During my time in hospital I didn't suffer much pain. I was medicated the first week in intensive care and after that I was drug free. What I do remember is being in a state of deep peace, a warm nurturing feeling.

I was growing more frustrated as I couldn't do many active things. I looked OK on the outside but I was physically weak and fragile on the inside and was very wary of doing too much. I was on the constant round of seeing doctors, specialists and physiotherapists, anyone who could help me improve my quality of life. Up to this point I had been focusing on conventional western medicine to help heal my physical body but I was starting to question myself, and my enquiry was taking me to the core of who I was, why I was here and what my purpose was in life. At the age of twenty four I left the security of the corporate world to embark on a journey into personal growth, meditation and spiritual development.

My osteopath evaluated me as a 26-year-old with the body of a 65-year-old in decline, and suggested I take up Taiji (Tai Chi). Initially it was another therapy to do and I just did it. But it all started to make sense. I realised that I could exercise, meditate and develop myself all at once. I realised from the first lesson that this is what I will do for the rest of my life. The gentle flowing movements brought an instant feeling of peace and this is what I had been trying to rediscover. Most importantly, I could do it. Yoga

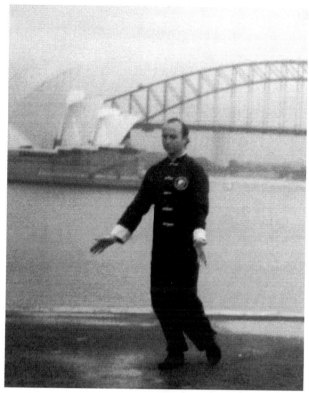

Sydney 1993

was too physical for me, I had limited movement in my legs and ankles and I couldn't sit cross-legged. Even standing without good supportive shoes was difficult. From the first Taiji class I felt at home. I remember looking around the class and thinking, "I could do this, I could be a Taiji instructor".

I always seemed to be the youngest in the class. I was 26 years old and after only a few months some of the ladies in my class would ask me to help them with their movements. After another year I became a class assistant and helped the instructors in the running of the class. I was a good student and I arranged my schedule so I would never miss a class. The group lesson and practice had a sense of community, it was non-competitive and everyone supported each other. My internal and external strength was slowly increasing and I felt very comfortable and natural in front of a group of students. I was starting to find purpose in my life. Over the next few years I was accepted as a trainee instructor and then appointed as a Taiji instructor with the Australian Academy of Tai Chi (AATC).

In 1990, at the age of 30, I learnt the Taiji Qigong Shibashi from Master Xia Shoude, a coach from the Beijing Institute of Physical Culture who had relocated to Sydney and was working for the AATC. Taiji Qigong Shibashi was a more recent development of the Chinese Healing Arts and was being widely promoted throughout the world in the late 1980s and early 1990s. Master Shoude was very dedicated and thorough in his instruction and produced detailed notes on the movements and their benefits. When you learn a new form it's always a bit overwhelming; there is so much to remember and the best way to learn is to teach.

Around that time an old friend had contacted me who was working at Sunnyhurst, a centre for the intellectually disabled. He heard that I was a Taiji instructor and invited me to come out and meet the guys and see if we could start a class. I had never had any experience in this area and had never met anyone with an intellectual disability. We had twenty in the class, so I played gentle relaxation music and commenced to teach them the Shibashi. To my amazement they loved it and were quite good. They invited me back the next week and I continued for eleven years. When my schedule became too busy, I handed the class over to one of the students who still runs the group, now twice a week. I taught them the Taiji Qigong Shibashi, but they taught me how to teach. Five years after starting the journey into the Chinese Healing Arts I committed myself to work full-time in spreading its benefits.

Many opportunities arose to work with different types of people. But I was mainly interested in working with people who would not have the opportunity to come into contact with this type of self-healing exercise. I was looking for challenges.

What I had been studying and teaching was called Taiji, and this had become a generalised term for Chinese relaxation exercises. The slow, gentle movements represented a choreographed martial art fighting sequence, a bit like shadow boxing with an imaginary opponent. The correct term is Taijiquan (Tai Chi Chuan) which translates to English as the Supreme Ultimate Fist. Taiji represents the Yin and Yang symbol and Quan means fist or boxing; it's one of the traditional Chinese internal martial arts.

As I was starting to work with groups of people in therapeutic communities I found the Taijiquan forms were not appropriate. Firstly, it took too long to learn. With regular practise it took a minimum of one year. Secondly, new students were starting at each session. At the drug and alcohol rehabilitation centres and prison groups, some would stay for one class and some would continue for a few months. I needed to make each session a session within itself, a mini-workshop enabling everyone to relieve stress and find inner peace. Also I didn't want to engage and direct the energy in martial arts techniques.

I developed the warm-up exercises as a dynamic meditation. It centred on intention, and focusing the mind on different parts of the body to gain a mind-body integration. This was followed by Daoist Yoga stretching exercises and a few of the Taiji Qigong Shibashi movements. To make it work I had to be consistent in creating a structure; the group sessions had to be at the same time and follow the same procedure. I had to be completely focused within myself to be in the present moment to hold the energy of the group, and to envelop the group with my energy or Qi. A question I'm often asked is, "Do I get much out of the class when I'm teaching?" I find the benefits are magnified many times as I'm completely in the moment while facilitating a class.

In 1995 I embarked on my first study tour of China with the AATC. It was a two-week tour with a large group and we visited cultural centres as well as historical Taijiquan and martial arts destinations. I was very excited to be in China. Taijiquan and Qigong were being very heavily promoted by the Chinese Government at that time, so we saw many demonstrations of different styles. What struck me most was the difference between the way the Chinese were doing it and the way we practised Taijiquan. Even though my basic movements were smooth and I understood the basic principles, the Chinese seemed to be more physical with larger, circular movements. Also there were no opportunities to stop, learn and absorb what I was seeing. I knew that I would have to return to China.

A few months after I returned from China I received a message from a Chinese couple, who wanted to meet me. They had seen me leading a demonstration in Chinatown earlier that year as a part of the Sydney Chinese New Year Celebrations. We met in a park near Chinatown. I saw a small group of Chinese people practising Taijiquan, they saw me and waved me over. I was introduced to Sifu, an honorary term for teacher. He gave a demonstration of Taijiquan and it was very impressive, much better than I had seen in China. He invited me to practise push hands with him, a two-person exercise of moving and harmonising the energy. I had little experience with push hands at that stage. He adjusted my technique a few times and we practised for about 10 minutes, finally he said "good", and gave me the thumbs up and the small group cheered and clapped.

They then grabbed my arm and whisked me off to a local restaurant where they had a table booked for Yum Cha. I was seated next to Sifu, and introduced to his wife, mother, brother and a few of their friends. He was a very proud man and radiated an amazing energy. He didn't speak English and his brother did the translating. Master William Ho was about 50 years old and had recently moved to Sydney from Taiwan. He was from a long family linage of Taijiquan Masters. After we finished eating he took me to a local Taijiquan class, and whilst sitting at the back he asked me my opinion on what the teacher was presenting and how the students were practising. He seemed to like my answers and gave me a big smile, said "Good" and gave me the thumbs up.

He invited me to train with him. I was teaching a lot of classes at that time, over twenty a week and we worked out on Tuesdays and Thursdays 6.30am to 8.30am at the spot in the park were we had met that day. It was traditional training one-on-one. Sifu knew two words in English, 'good' and 'no good'. He knew the exact movements for every posture and we would practise the martial art fighting sequence for every movement. After a few months when I had learnt the basic Yang Style Taijiquan and push hands techniques he asked me if I would like for him to become my Master. A party was arranged in a large Chinese restaurant and I became initiated as Master Ho's first student, like his first son. Master Ho didn't have any children of his own and was completely dedicated to teaching traditional Chinese martial arts. I held an honoured position and the other students held me in high regard. I would help teach the new students and lead the practice sessions.

By the end of 1995 I resigned from the AATC. After coming back from China six months earlier my Taijiquan had turned full circle. When you are ready the Master will appear. With clear intention the universe seems to manifest the right people at the right time.

My physical body and energy were becoming stronger, but my feet and legs would still ache. Over the years I had taken advice from doctors, physiotherapists, osteopaths, acupuncturists, meditation masters, yoga teachers, and Taijiquan and Qigong masters on the best way to manage my condition. In time we become our own best doctor by learning what works best for us. Sometimes I would need rest and other times the right stretch would relieve pain, but what I observed was the relationship between my mind and my body. When my mind was in a calm, relaxed state without physical or emotional desires my body felt light and agile without any pain. Teaching became a passion. I seemed to step outside of myself when I was with a group. The energy would flow through me into the group. I felt physically, emotionally and spiritually strong.

In 1994, before resigning from the AATC, I met Qigong Grand Master Jack Lim and attended a few of his workshops. He had a different approach from the mainly martial teachers that I had met up to this stage. Jack would talk about the relationship between our self, nature and the universe. He would teach different movements and meditations to harmonise the energy channels or meridians, bringing about a state of inner peace and allowing a natural healing to occur. In 1996, after I had resigned from the AATC, I became Qigong Grand Master Jack Lim's assistant and helped him when he was in Sydney at the Mind, Body, Spirit Festivals and conducting workshops. Jack was unique as he was born and raised in Australia before spending 25 years in China studying Qigong. He was able to translate the meaning and essence of the Chinese Healing Arts into terms that I could understand and also guide me to a deeper understanding of the Qi energy and myself. He would tell me about the sacred mountains, the rich culture of the Chinese people and the study tours he lead there.

I was receiving very positive feedback from the students in my classes – their comments were similar, mainly about how clarity of mind would improve many aspects of their lives. These comments were coming from different types of people, from ladies in their 80s to 20-year-old recovering drug addicts, inmates in prisons, business executives, health care workers and therapists, even high school students. Everyone was seeking ways of relieving stress, of bringing the mind and body into balance and discovering inner peace.

The mid-1990s was a huge growth period internationally for the Chinese Healing Arts. Many research projects and articles were published on the benefits of practising these ancient arts. The Energy Field' was a gathering of all the different schools in Sydney in a non-competitive environment, to give demonstrations and showcase their styles. I was involved with Master Ho and Ancestral Tai Chi. At the 1997 event I met John Dolic, the publisher of Qigong Chinese Health Magazine and a practitioner of Chinese Medicine and teacher of Qigong and Wushu. I arranged a meeting with John and he agreed to teach me the Ba Duan Jin (Eight Pieces of Brocade). He taught it to me at his clinic with direct reference to meridian charts, describing how the exercise worked in stimulating the different energy channels and its basic Traditional Chinese Medicine theory. I started teaching this to all my groups after the warm-up as a way of purging the meridians. John would also talk about his time in China studying and the different Masters he had learnt from.

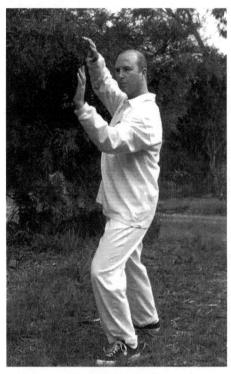 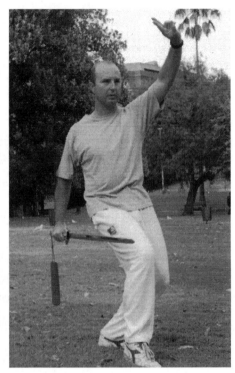

Sydney 1996   Sydney 1997

I had read about Taijiquan competitions in China and the US and when the opportunity arose to compete in one of the earliest events in 1998 in Sydney, I decided to enter with three of Master Ho's students. Sifu trained us very hard, practising the 24 movement Yang Style, the 32 movement Straight Sword, push hand techniques and standing Qigong to strengthen our Qi. There is a lot of controversy between the old traditional styles and the newer styles sanctioned by the Chinese Government and this was evident when the head judge told me we weren't doing it right. I was congratulated by the other judges and won first prize in the open 32 Movement Straight Taijquan Sword. I was later invited to become a judge in the 2000 and 2001 Peaceful Challenge Australian Tai Chi Titles.

Qigong Grand Master Jack Lim told me about the 4th World Conference on Medical Qigong to be held in Beijing, China in 1998. Jack was a Standing Council Member of this association and was not attending so he suggested that I go, as it would be a great opportunity to meet other Qigong practitioners. When the master gives an order you just do it. I was very pleased to be returning to China. There were 600 people in attendance from most areas around the world. I didn't know anyone, but Jack had phoned the chairperson, Professor Feng Lida, to personally introduce me to the world community. I attended lectures presented by professors and doctors from Qigong research departments of major universities in China, Japan and Korea which were using modern scientific devises to show the existence of Qi and how it healed, including many clinical cases. I also attended workshops by professors and masters which included theory and specific Qigong training methods. All my previous years of training were coming to fruition as I realised that I knew more than I thought I did.

I spent a lot of my spare time with Professor Jerry Alan Johnson, an American Qigong Grand Master who was writing a series of Medical

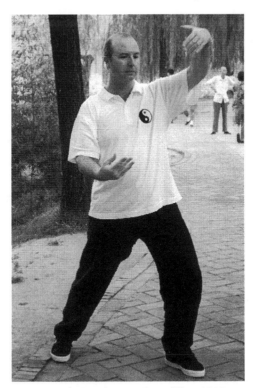

Purple Bamboo Park, Beijing 1998

Qigong books. Jerry started his journey with the martial arts, then studied Traditional Chinese Medicine, Qigong and Daoist Mysticism. I liked his direct no-nonsense approach. We shared many ideas and had a similar understanding.

What he told me had a big influence on the next stage of my journey. He explained his understanding of the progression of developing yourself within the Chinese Healing Arts. We generally start with the martial forms of Qigong. Becoming the warrior when we are younger shows us a way of learning discipline and structure, and building the Qi. From the warrior we start to enquire and question ourself and become the scholar and study the classics on medicine, art, philosophy and spirituality. This leads us to the healer, healing ourself both physically and emotionally, awakening spiritually and healing others as a way of gaining merit for the negative karma accumulated from the warrior. This leads us to become one with the universe, the Dao, God or whatever your understanding of the divine.

I have told this story many times, thank you Jerry, mainly to my groups in rehabilitation programs. I explain that you don't want to be the warrior when you are 65 years of age, still fighting in the streets for your existence. By that age we should have moved through life, learning from our adventures and growing and developing to become a valuable member of the community.

My Taijiquan and Qigong training, at this stage being twelve years, plus the last ten years, have fully enveloped my life. However, by meeting other practitioners at the conference and being exposed to the world stage I realised that I was still in the early stages of this journey into the Chinese Healing Arts. I knew when I started that it would take a long time; the Chinese have a word for this, Gong Fu (Kung Fu) which translates to skill and time. It takes time to acquire a skill; there is Gong Fu in gaining skills in all areas of life. It's important to take your time, set your destination and work towards it and factor in the time it's going to take to arrive there. It's like the foundations of a bridge which need to be solidly grounded in the earth to enable people to cross safely.

I developed the Qigong warm-up, Ba Duan Jin, and Taiji Qigong Shibashi followed by sitting meditation as my core practices. I then made my first VHS video 'Qigong – The Art of Life' in 1999, followed by the DVD in 2003 and now the Book/DVD The Art of Life in 2010.

I was mainly interested in teaching Qigong and meditation. I did have a few groups to whom I would teach Taijiquan, including the sword, but I found that it would generate a different kind of energy. To teach it correctly the martial applications and push hand techniques had to be practised. There were usually questions and some discussion regarding martial techniques. I never had a great interest in the martial arts; my journey into Taijiquan was mainly to regain strength and discover the inner peace that I experienced when I had that near-death experience. Jerry's story was making sense and it was time to give away the warrior. By 2002 I had stopped teaching and practising Taijiquan and stepped aside from my commitment with Master Ho.

As the second millennium was drawing to a close my journey was now taking me to the source, returning to China and travelling to India. It was now time to Absorb the Essence.

TO BE CONTINUED…

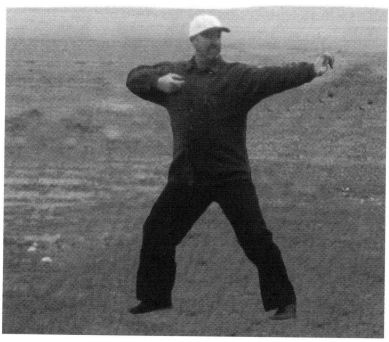

Grasslands, Inner Mongolia 2002

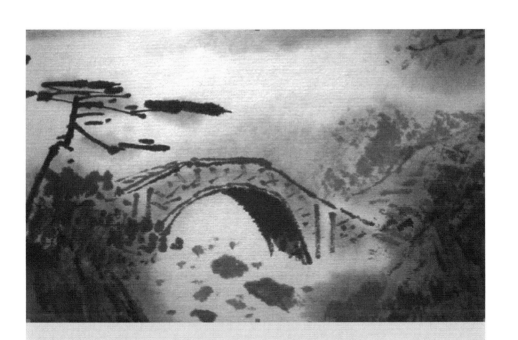

Chapter 5

The Art of Practice

The Art of Life

The Art of Practice

To get the most out of your practice there are a few basic principles that apply to the styles of Qigong presented in this book.

Time of day to practise

Generally, you can practise Qigong at any time of the day, so choose a time that best suits you. Remember, we are creatures of habit and you will benefit more if you practise at the same time on each practice day. Some styles of Qigong are best practised at a particular time and sometimes facing a certain direction. In time you will find the best time that suits you.

Exercising in the early morning and late afternoon, when the sun rises and sets, is a very powerful time as it's a natural transition between dark coolness of night (Yin) and the bright warmth of day (Yang). It's important not to look directly into the sun in the early morning or late afternoon as this can cause damage to your eyes. The setting of the sun and transition between Yang and Yin is a time when nature has a great influence on your body. You might notice that birds are very active at this time of the day, as they are in the morning.

I am often asked by new students if it's best to practise with the eyes open or closed, and what does one look at when practising. It may be easier to concentrate when the eyes are closed as we are not distracted by things around us, but the general rule with Qigong is to have the eyes open when moving, looking to the distance but not really looking. Your awareness is on the external (Yang) when the eyes are open and you can absorb the energy or Qi from the environment and universe. It's OK to momentarily close the eyes but it's important to keep them open – not too wide, and relaxed. When practising Qigong meditation or Neigong the eyes are closed as your awareness is now on the internal (Yin).

As a rule, you should not exercise on a full or empty stomach. Instead of eating breakfast, consume liquids as they stimulate stomach-intestine movement which acts as an internal massage. Warm or room temperature water is the best with a slice of lemon. Cold water from the fridge interferes with Qi circulation.

Qigong exercise in the evenings is a way to free your mind and body from the burdens of a busy day and a way of processing the events of the day and letting things go, physically and emotionally. Students often comment on how they get their best night's sleep after attending class. You will then be able to sleep more quietly and recover more fully because the body begins its recovery during Qigong and this continues during sleep.

"When I practise my Qigong in the evening, I sleep much better. Therefore I have more energy the next day." Cherel Waters

We are all a bit different. I wouldn't advise that you practise immediately before going to sleep as it stimulates your energy and may disrupt your sleep. But a few students have told me that when they haven't been able to sleep they get up and practise which calms their mind and body. They then have a restful sleep.

Eating and drinking

For Qigong exercise you need a clear head. Beverages such as alcohol, tea and coffee affect concentration and body functions and if you are not calm and relaxed you will not feel the full benefits of Qigong exercise. It's best to avoid drinking cold fluids during or immediately after practice as this interferes with Qi circulation.

When I was training with Master Ho we began early in the morning at 6.30am and he would take my pulse before and after practice. A few times he became very concerned as my heart rate and organ functions were erratic. He watched me very closely, my movements were slow and smooth and my breath deep and even. After a lot of questions I told him I had a strong espresso coffee half an hour before we started. I have now changed my morning routine and only have warm water or green tea.

Avoid exercising on either an empty stomach or after a full meal. Being distracted by hunger will not help your mental focus so if you are hungry, have something light to eat or something to drink. A full stomach interferes with Qi circulation. The Qi is diverted into the digestive system as stomach juices increase and stomach-intestinal movements occur, leaving very little Qi to circulate elsewhere.

When not to exercise

When we exercise we absorb the good influences from nature and the macrocosm. Similarly, we absorb the influences from turbulent weather conditions. Therefore, it is not good to practise Qigong during bad weather, heavy fog, extreme heat, before or during a thunderstorm, on excessively windy days, or during lunar or solar eclipses. Exercise can begin again when nature is balanced.

Menstruation and pregnancy

Basic Qigong is good to practise during menstruation and pregnancy as it will improve the circulation of Qi, blood and other body fluids.

Women who are menstruating should pay attention to the effects of Qigong exercise. If the exercise produces a negative effect, stop immediately and continue when feeling better.

Special care is also required during pregnancy. Each woman's pregnancy is different, and it is recommended that the expectant mother consult her primary care provider as well as a qualified and experienced Qigong teacher.

> *"I attended Simon's week-long retreat during my pregnancy and experienced a great release of muscle tension particularly in my arms and shoulders. I also found the meditation that followed the Qigong practice easy to do even though I had never meditated before. It was a very pleasurable experience."* Jessica Henley

Where to practise

Qigong can be practised anywhere but some places are better than others. It's best to be undisturbed during Qigong practice to help maintain a concentrated mind. The best places are in nature in the open air where the Heaven (Yang) and Earth (Yin) Qi are most abundant such as in the mountains, beside a waterfall or by the ocean. Near a waterfall or by the ocean is excellent because moving water generates lots of Qi.

If you are practising indoors, try to find a quiet and peaceful space away from draughts, with natural light and fresh air. Avoid excessive noise, TV sets and computers and turn off your mobile phone or set it to silent.

The proximity of some plants should also be avoided. The Oleander plant for example, is known to be poisonous and has a very tense Qi. As you practise you will learn which plants feel relaxing and harmonious. Lovely flowers and large old trees are ideal.

What to wear

There are no rules regarding clothing but since relaxation is important in Qigong try to wear loose comfortable clothing, ideally made of natural fibres such as cotton or silk.

If you are limited in what you can wear, for example if you are at work, loosen your collar and tie, your belt/waistband and remove uncomfortable or high heel shoes. It's important that you wear flat soled shoes or even bare feet are OK. I always wear soft sports shoes as I damaged my feet and ankles a long time ago and I find wearing shoes gives me a bit more support. It's a personal preference. There are many light, soft shoes around today.

Whatever clothing you choose to wear it should not be tight around the waist because the Qi needs to flow easily. Preferably, remove watches and bracelets as they restrict the flow of Qi through the wrist.

If it is chilly, dress appropriately. Feeling cold during a Qigong session can decrease the effectiveness of the exercises particularly if your hands, belly and back are cold. Chilling your kidneys severely restricts your Qi circulation. I often start my practice on colder mornings with gloves, hat and a warm jacket and I can always take them off.

How long to practise

The benefits that are gained from Qigong are proportional to the amount of practice. For beginners, an exercise period of 15 to 30 minutes daily is recommended in order to relax the body and mind and feel the Qi. It is only when the body's carriage is regulated according to Qigong principles that the Qi will flow easily and the benefits of Qigong realised. If you can achieve 30 minutes twice a day, you will notice a marked increase in vitality and peace within a few weeks. If you have major health issues and can manage a couple of hours per day you will soon see a radical improvement in your health and wellbeing. Regardless of your state of health when you begin, any amount of regular practice will improve how you feel.

> *"I have practised Qigong every day for sixteen years. It helps bring me right into the present moment with a feeling of immense serenity. Each year my health has improved and whenever I experience a set-back, gentle Qigong is always there to help me."* Joan Downey

> *"Over the last few years I have been practising five to six times per week. I am in my 80th year and have gone from wearing a hinged metal knee brace to wearing no brace at all. My knee still creaks but is no longer painful and range of movement is barely restricted."* Shirley Chittick

How long does the effect of Qigong exercise last?

Qigong works because the Qi is brought into order and the mind, body and spirit are in harmony. This harmony can be disturbed by arguing, getting excited or annoyed, engaging in strenuous physical activity, eating excessively, and even going to the toilet. If possible, use the toilet beforehand rather than after Qigong exercise because urination and defecation bring the Qi into definite motion.

I often tell my students after a Qigong class that if they have driven a car to get to the class try not to play the radio when they leave because all the senses have been enhanced and body functions are in harmony. In the quietness and stillness you may get good ideas, solve some problems, or if you are with friends you might have some amazing conversations. Look at the beauty of the sky, trees, the divine in all living things. I love to look at clouds. It's a creative time, so use it wisely and the Qi will be with you longer. The more you cultivate your Qi the more in harmony with the universe you will be, improving all aspects of your life.

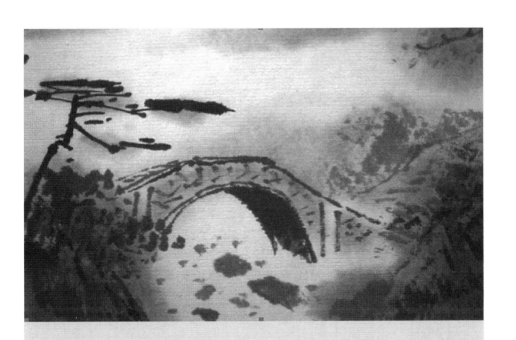

Chapter 6

Qigong Warm-up

The Art of Life

Qigong warm-up

There are many ways of preparing for Qigong practice. Some parts of the warm-up were taught to me, some I observed by watching people practising in parks in China, and other parts I have developed from my own practice.

The warm-up is not only a way of preparing the mind and body for the Qigong movements that come later, it's also very good exercise. Physically, when we loosen and rotate the joints, we exercise the ligaments and tendons, as well as the membranes which secrete synovial fluid to lubricate the joints. This can benefit many arthritic conditions. Energetically, we clear stagnant energy (Qi) that can accumulate around the joints. According to Traditional Chinese Medicine (TCM), the Qi draws the blood through the body. So when we stimulate the Qi circulation we also stimulate the blood circulation.

It's also very important to focus your awareness, like the light of a torch, on each part of the body as we are exercising it, from head to toe. Through this active meditation we consciously awaken the body by feeling and seeing what we are doing.

Generally, when we have finished the warm-up, we feel warm, tingling and awake.

Posture and breathing

During the warm-up and practice we first concentrate on the body posture. In either a standing or sitting position, keep the spine upright and let the muscles and flesh relax around the skeleton. The movements of Qigong help clear the energy blockages in our body. Also known as guiding Qi, movements will become slow, soft and smooth with regular practice. Then we can concentrate on the breath.

There are a number of different breathing patterns for different styles of Qigong. For the styles presented here, we will breathe in and out through the nose to the abdominal area, slowly, deeply and deliberately. When we breathe in, the abdomen gently expands and when breathing out, it gently contracts. This is known as natural breathing. In time, the breath will naturally coordinate with the movements, helping the mind to focus and allowing a fusion between mind, body and breath.

The practice of Qigong should become a pleasurable experience and when you are practising correctly, a gentle, natural smile will permeate throughout the whole body, from the heart through every cell. As Qigong Grand Master Jack Lim often told me, you can tell if a student has understood a lesson, not by his performance of the movements, but by the smile at the end of the class.

Basic stance

Stand with feet parallel, shoulder-width apart, as if standing on train tracks. Knees are slightly off lock. Let your weight sink into your legs, feet and into the ground. Keep the coccyx or tail bone slightly tucked in, chest relaxed, and the back straight. Hold your arms away from the body, fingers open and relaxed pointing to the earth, palms facing the body.

Please note that the images are mirrored for the reader; just follow in the same direction.

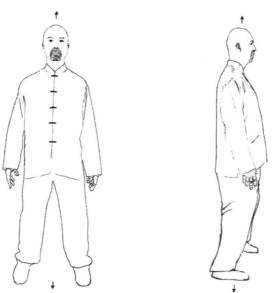

With the chin slightly tucked in and the top of the head (Bai Hui point) reaching to the sky as if a silken cord attached to it is lifting the whole body, light the Hui Yin by gently squeezing the pelvic floor. Relax your eyes and face and look out into the distance. Keeping your jaw relaxed, place the tip of your tongue on the top palate of your mouth, just behind the front teeth. Breathe in and out through the nose. When breathing in, let the abdomen push out slightly and as the breath comes out, let the abdomen contract. Just relax, letting the whole body breathe.

With the eyes closed, allow the breath to become smooth and even, and let your mind rest. After a few breaths, concentrate on the out-breath, relaxing from the top of the head to the soles of the feet. Just relax down through the body on the out-breath. After a few more breaths, let the knees and hips sink a bit closer to the ground and feel the pressure go into the feet. Like a tree, follow the roots from the soles of your feet deeply into the ground. As you let the breath out, relax down through the body into the ground, letting the stress and tension of the body dissolve into the earth.

After another few breaths, with your awareness, push up the spine one vertebra at a time, checking that the chin tucks in and letting the head pull away from the body. We seem to stand taller as the top of the head reaches up and touches the sky. Stay in this posture for a few breaths, feeling the peace. With your eyes gradually opening, look out into the distance.

The warm-up movements

Shoulder rolls

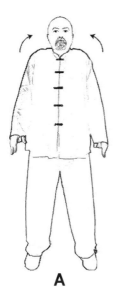 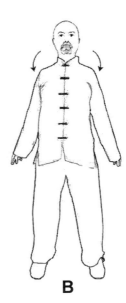

A   Lift the shoulders and start to rotate them backwards.

B   After about four to six rotations, reverse, gradually increasing your range of movement.

Wrist rotations

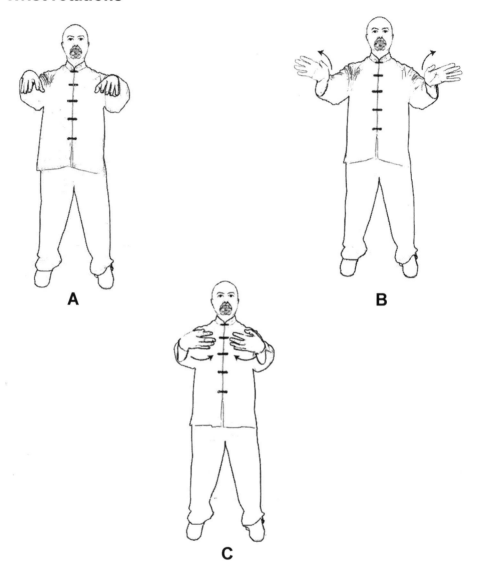

A   Slowly raise the arms to shoulder height.

B   Rotate the wrists, as though the fingers are drawing circles in the air. Feel and see the movement of the wrist.

C   After about 4 to 6 rotations stop and come back the other way, gradually increasing your range of movement.

Arm and chest stretch

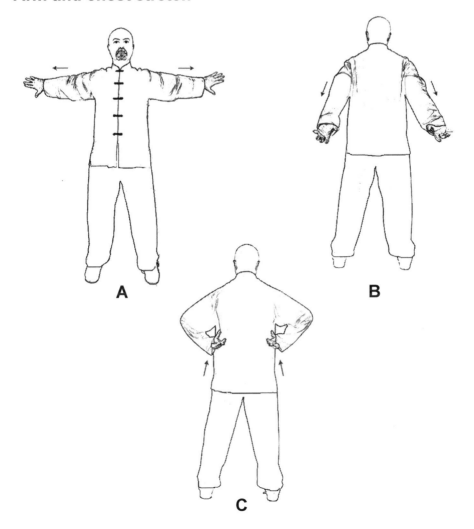

A
B
C

A With your arms still in front of the body, turn your palms out and push to the sides, seeing your chest and rib cage open. Push back and stretch back as far as comfortable.

B Turn your palms up, bend the elbows and bring hands to the front of body brushing by the waist. Repeat 4 times, similar to swimming breaststroke.

C Then repeat 4 times in the opposite direction: with palms up, hands brush by your waist and stretch behind, slowly rotate palms and bring arms in front of body. This movement exercises the chest, shoulders, elbows and wrists.

Body roll

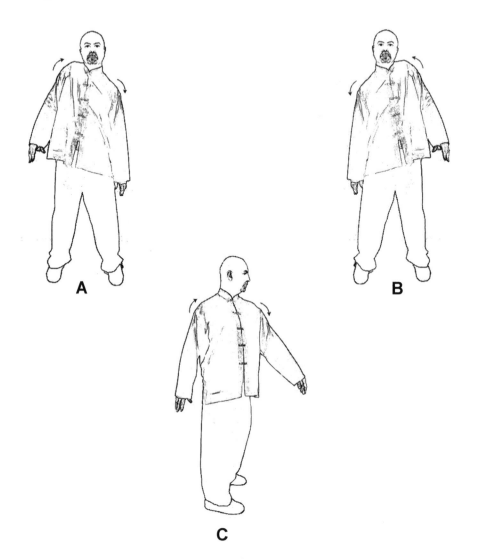

A Let your arms slowly descend to your sides. Slowly roll one shoulder and then the other, like swimming backwards. With your awareness, feel the motion massage around your shoulders, your chest, around the back of your shoulders and your abdomen, also massaging your back over the kidney area.

B, C After about 8 rotations, stop and come back the other way, and feel the internal massaging.

Hip rotations

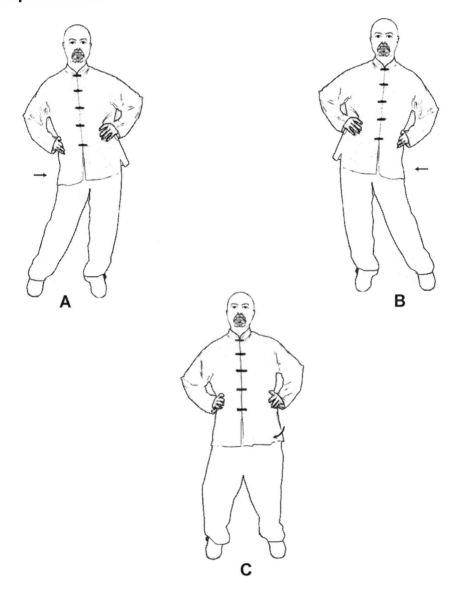

A, B   Place your hands on your waist and start to move your hips from side to side. Relax and feel the movement of the hips.

C   After about three movements to each side, start to move the hips in a circle, gradually increasing your range of movement. Follow the spiralling movement up the spine to the top of your head. Feel and see the movement of the hips. After about 6 rotations, stop and come back the other way.

Walking and massaging the feet

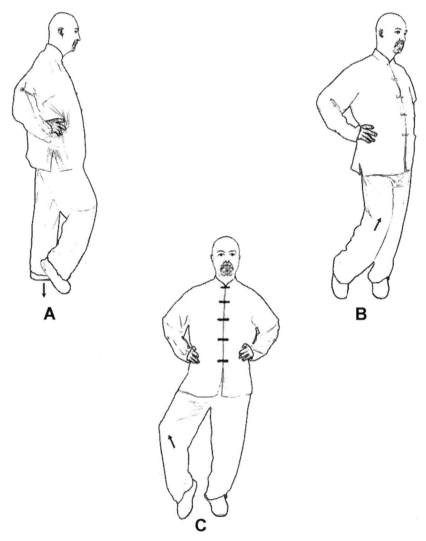

A Stand with your feet closer together, walking on the spot. Push firmly
   from the toe to the heel six times to each side, letting the weight of the
   body massage the feet. Feel and see the tendons, muscles and joints of
   the feet.

B Turn and twist while moving your knee across the body, massaging
   the inside of the foot on the floor towards the big toe. Repeat about 6
   times to each side.

C Stop and push to the outside of the foot, massaging towards the small
   toe, 6 to each side. Relax, feel and see the movement of the foot.

Foot, leg and hip rotation

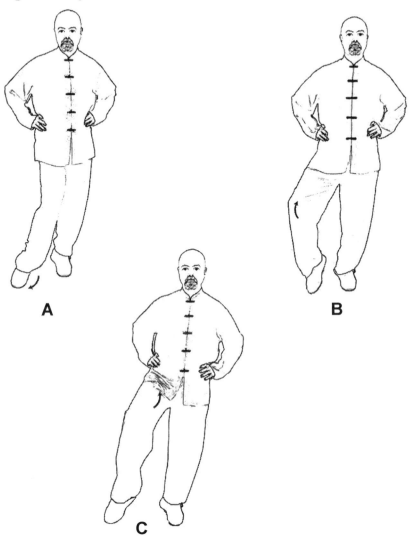

A

B

C

A, B, Standing on your right leg, place the tip of the left big toe on the
C ground and start to rotate, using your awareness to feel the massage
around your toes and foot. See your ankle rotating and the knee
rotating, right up to your hip. Moving the whole leg together, relax,
feel and see the movement of the leg. Stop and come back the other
way, gradually increasing the range of movement.

Repeat the same process for your right leg and then shake out your legs,
feeling the flow of blood and Qi.

Hand and wrist shaking

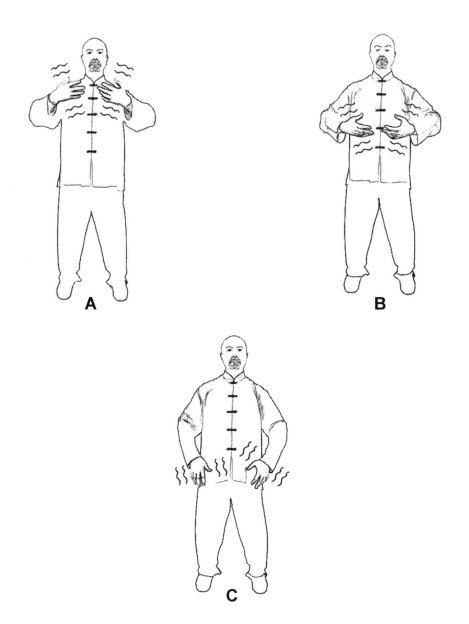

A, B, Shake your hands, up and down about 6 times, loosening the hands.
C

Hand stretching

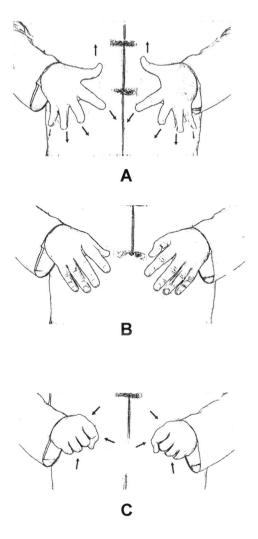

A, B   Extend the hands, stretching all the fingers. It's important not to hold the movement – extend and relax, 6 times.

C   Then clench the fists – again, don't hold. Clench and relax, 6 times.

With the palms up, roll the fingers, starting with the small finger, into a fist and clench with your thumb on outside, 6 times, concentrating on the hands. Stop and roll into a fist the other way, index finger first, 6 times. Again, shake the hands up and down, also moving the knees up and down as you shake the whole body.

Body swings

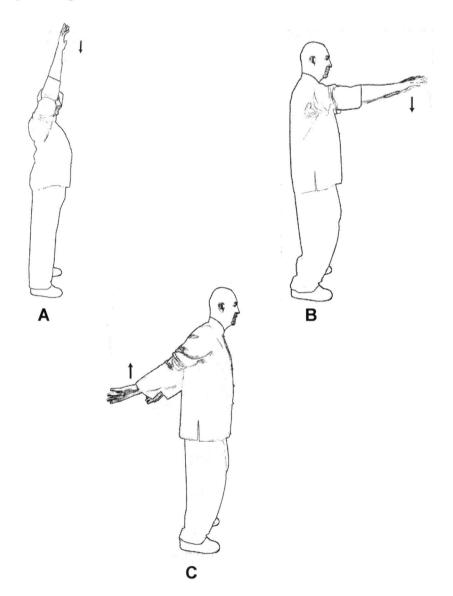

A

B

C

A, B, With the feet parallel and arms above the head, swing the arms
C down, sinking the knees at the same time. Let the whole body swing, keep the back straight and head upright. With your awareness, relax the shoulder and hips, elbows and knees, wrists and ankles, hands and feet. Do this for about 12 swings. This helps strengthen the whole body and is good for the blood circulation.

Swinging arms

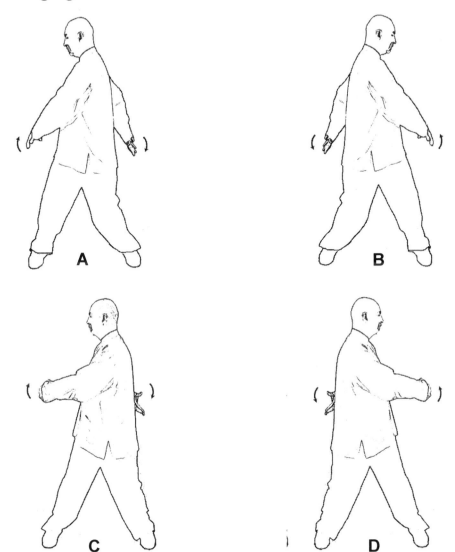

A, B Step out to a wider horse-riding stance. With the legs grounded firmly, the arms relaxed, let your arms swing out, turning from the waist. Let the arms slap across the body, massaging around the waist and hips.

C, D Let your arms swing higher, massaging around the kidneys and finally, still higher as one swinging arm taps the shoulder while the other taps the kidneys. Do this 12 times. This helps loosen and strengthen the back and helps massage the internal organs.

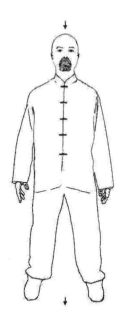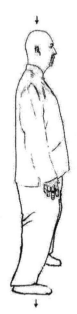

After the swinging exercises, stand in the basic stance and relax from the top of your head down to your hands and down to your feet, relax down through the body on the out breath for a few minutes.

We are now ready to practise our Qigong.

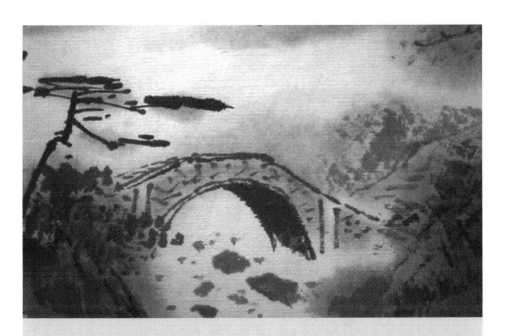

Chapter 7

Ba Duan Jin
Eight Method Essence Standing

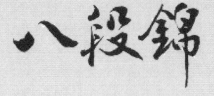

The Art of Life

Ba Duan Jin Eight Method Essence Standing

Translating to 'Eight Method Essence', Ba Duan Jin has a few different names outside of China such as the Eight Pieces of Brocade, the Eight Golden Treasures, the Eight Pieces of Silk and many others. It is one of the most renowned and widely practised forms of Qigong in China and known throughout the world by martial artists, Tai Chi groups, Qigong and Traditional Chinese Medicine (TCM) practitioners for its healing benefits. Its origin traces back to ancient times. History books suggest that the legendary Yeuh Fei 1100AD (Sung Dynasty), a Chinese General, was an early proponent, and the first to train his troops in Martial Arts (Wushu) and the therapeutic, self-healing Standing Ba Duan Jin. There are variations of the Ba Duan Jin, but they all follow the same principle.

Also known as Taoist Yoga, in traditional terms, it is a Wei Dan Gong style of Qigong which translates to 'external elixir training'. The physical stretching movements stimulate the flow of Qi through the organ meridians as they increase strength and flexibility of the whole body.

Meridians

While Western medicine recognises only three circulatory networks in the human body – the nervous system, the lymphatic system and the blood vessels – Traditional Chinese Medicine includes a fourth system: the energy network of meridians. Meridians are pathways or channels which transport Qi through the whole body ensuring the tissues and organs are supplied with fluids and nutrients. They are all interconnected and form a network to connect the internal organs to external parts of the body.

Meridian lines cannot be seen or felt like other systems in the body such as the circulatory or nervous system. When a person is in good (balanced) health, their meridian lines will be open and clear of blockages. Qi can then flow smoothly.

These meridian lines can be associated with the functioning of the body's internal organs. The health of an organ is affected by the corresponding meridian and has a direct impact on the strength and energy of the meridian. If these organs function abnormally, the energy will stagnate in the meridians and cause illness. To return to good health the blockage must be released and the flow of energy normalised.

There are 12 known meridians, or rivers of energy, that flow through the body:

1. Triple Heater (Sanjao) meridian
2. Lung meridian
3. Large intestine meridian
4. Spleen meridian
5. Stomach meridian
6. Liver meridian
7. Gall bladder meridian
8. Kidney meridian
9. Bladder meridian
10. Heart meridian
11. Small intestine meridian
12. Pericardium meridian

The Meridian Cycle

Meridians are classified as Yin or Yang depending on which way they flow on the surface of the body. Yang energy flows from the sun, and Yang meridians run from the fingers to the face or from the face to the feet. Yin energy, from the earth, flows from the feet to the torso, and from the torso along the inside of the arms to the fingertips. Since the meridian flow is continuous and unbroken, the energy flows in one direction, and from one meridian to another in a well determined order. Since there is no beginning or end to this flow, the order can be represented as a wheel. The flow around the wheel follows the meridian lines on the body in this order:
- from torso to fingertip (along inside of arm – Yin)
- from fingertip to face (along outside/back of arm – Yang)
- from face to feet (along outside of leg – Yang)
- from feet to torso (along inside of the leg – Yin)

Preparation

Stand with feet together, eyes closed, chin tucked slightly in, as though a silken cord is pulling the head towards the sky, gently extending the spine. Keep the tip of tongue on the top palate of the mouth just behind the teeth. Breathe in and out naturally through the nose. Allow the breath to become smooth and even and the mind to relax.

Relax and feel. When you first start to practise Ba Duan Jin, you may feel different sensations in different parts of your body. Warmth and a tingling sensation in the hands, fingers, and other areas of your body are common. It's generally a sign that the Qi and blood are flowing through the energy channels, or meridians, clearing blockages. With regular practise, these sensations will ease. Between each section of the Ba Duan Jin, relax and feel as a way of monitoring your own energy system. A clear and peaceful mind is another good sign that the Qigong is flowing naturally and the mind is not detecting any imbalances. With regular practise, it's best to feel nothing or 'nothingness'.

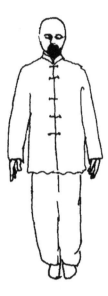

Please note that the images are mirrored for the reader; just follow in the same direction.

First Piece - Regulating the Sanjiao Channel

This translates to regulating the 'Triple Heater' or 'Energiser'.

According to Traditional Chinese Medicine (TCM), the Upper Heater relates to the organs above the diaphragm including the thorax, heart and lung, and aids the respiratory system of the body and heats up the air. The Upper Heater helps maintain the ability to absorb essence from the air and the universe.

The Middle Heater, located between the diaphragm and the navel, relates to the upper abdomen, the spleen, pancreas, stomach, liver, gall bladder and the small intestine. The Middle Heater functions like the oven of the body, heating the liquids and solids, and aiding in their digestion. The Middle Heater promotes the absorption of essence from foods.

The Lower Heater, below the navel, relates to the lower abdomen, kidneys, bladder and large intestine, and assists the elimination system of the body, also by heating up the solids and fluids.

The Sanjiao Channel runs up the outside of the arm from the tip of the outside of the ring finger to the wrist, up to the elbow and shoulder, up the neck to underneath the ear, circles the ear and finishes at the eyebrow.

Sanjiao Channel (Triple Heater)

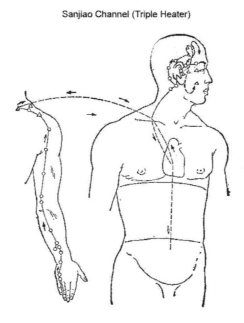

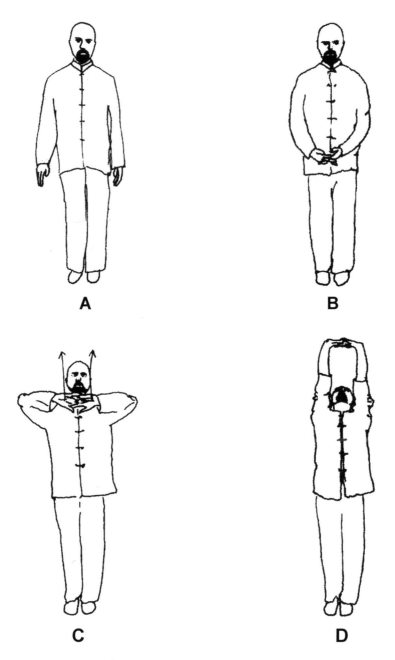

A, B Stand in the basic stance, breathe in, interlock the fingers in front of the navel and then pause on the out breath.

C, D Breathe in, bring hands up to chest level, and look up as you turn the hands palm upwards, still interlocked, and push to the sky.

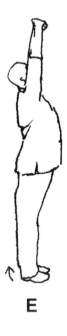

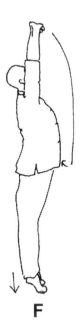

E   **F**

E, F At the same time push the legs down into the earth and go up on the toes (stimulating the Sanjiao Channel). Breathe out, lower the weight onto the heels and bring the hands straight down the front of the body, turning in a circle.

B End with hands palm up at navel at the starting position. Keep the legs straight.

Repeat 8 times.

A Stand, arms by the side of the body, feet together and close the eyes. Relax and feel.

Second Piece – Regulating the Lung and Large Intestine Channels

The main purpose of the lungs is to breathe in fresh air (oxygen) and expel waste gas (carbon dioxide), thereby helping the body's metabolism to function smoothly. According to TCM, the lungs operate the Qi of the whole body. Essence is absorbed from the universe through the nose into the lungs and spread throughout the whole body.

The Lung Channel (Yin) originates in the middle portion of the body, and runs downwards connecting with the large intestine. It then turns and passes through the diaphragm to connect with the lungs. This channel branches out from the armpit and runs down the inside of the arm to the outside of the thumb.

Another branch emerges from the back of the wrist and ends at the tip of the index finger to connect with the Large Intestine Channel.

The Large Intestine Channel (Yang) originates from the outside of the index finger through the Hegu, or tiger's mouth which is between the thumb and index finger, then along the outside of the arm to the shoulder, to the neck and finishes on the opposite side of the face near the nose and cheek bone.

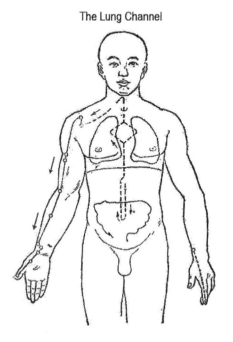

The Lung Channel

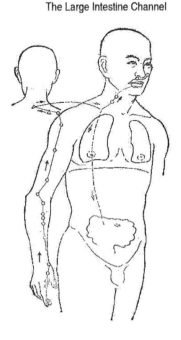

The Large Intestine Channel

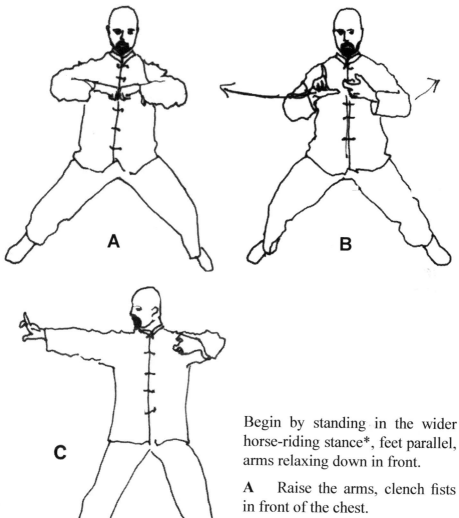

Begin by standing in the wider horse-riding stance*, feet parallel, arms relaxing down in front.

A   Raise the arms, clench fists in front of the chest.

B   With the left hand, open the tiger's mouth – extend thumb and index finger to form a right angle. With the right hand, close tiger's mouth – bend second knuckle of index finger, keeping thumb down.

C, D Extend the elbows horizontally, pull both arms back, and whilst breathing in stretch the left arm straight to the side with eyes focused over extended index finger. Keep the right arm bent, and elbow level with the shoulder. Stretch across your chest as if pulling back on a bow (stimulating the Lung and Large Intestine channels) and 'release the arrow' from the right hand.

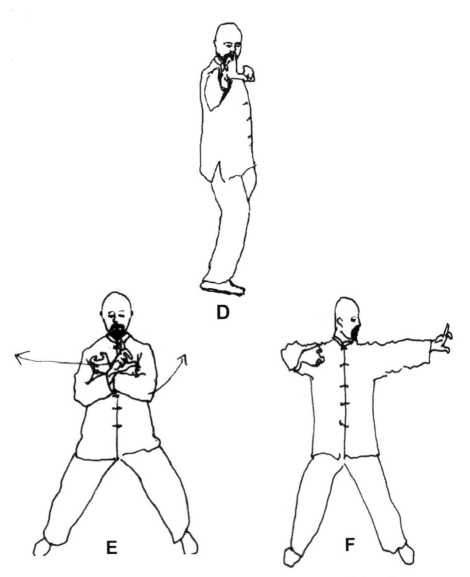

E, F Breathe out, bring the hands back to the centre of the chest, reverse hand positions and repeat on opposite side.

Repeat 4 times to each side.

Return to basic stance, arms down by your sides, feet together and close the eyes. Relax and feel.

* All movements using the horse-riding stance help stimulate the Kidney Channel.

Third Piece - Regulating the Spleen and Stomach Channels

The spleen is located on the left side of the abdominal area and is the main organ of the digestive system in TCM. The functions of the pancreas and the mouth also relate to the spleen which, according to TCM, is where food and fluids enter the body. The stomach digests the food, sending solids and fluids downward, while the essence is sent up to the spleen. The spleen transforms this essence and distributes it to the rest of the body.

The Spleen Channel (Yin) originates from the outside of the big toe, to the ankle, and rises up the inside of the leg to the hip, through the abdomen to the chest. The Stomach Channel (Yang) originates from beneath the eye, down to the corner of the mouth, around the jaw, and descends down the neck to the nipple, and down the centre of the body to the pubic bone. From the hip, it continues down the front of the leg, passing the knee, through the middle of the front of the ankle, and finishing on the outside of the second toe.

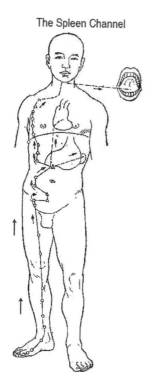

The Spleen Channel

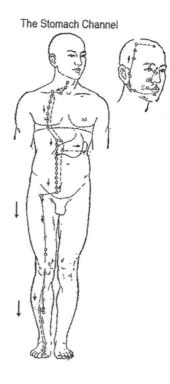

The Stomach Channel

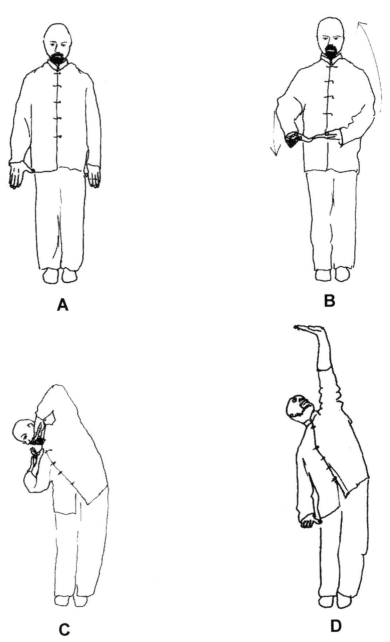

A

B

C

D

A   Stand with feet together. With the left hand, open tiger's mouth keeping the other fingers flat and together (not in a fist as in Second Piece). With the right hand, close tiger's mouth keeping fingers and thumb out flat and together.

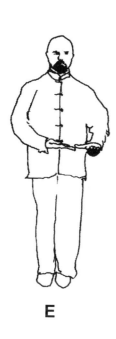

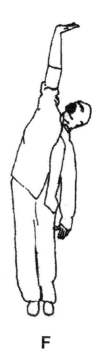

E   **F**

B, C, Leaning slightly to the left, push the left hand down as you push the
D   right hand up, breathing in. Check that the hand pushing down has
the fingers pointing forward in the same direction as the feet. The
hand pushing up should have fingers pointing horizontally 90° to the
downward pushing hand (stimulating the Lung and Large Intestine
Channels).

E, F Breathing out, turn top hand palm inwards and let it fall down in front
of the body, then place both arms at the side of the body. Reverse
hand positions and repeat on opposite side.

Repeat 4 times to each side.

Return to basic stance – stand, arms at the sides, feet together and close the
eyes. Relax and feel.

Fourth Piece - Regulating the Liver and Gall Bladder Channels

The liver helps to cleanse the blood. TCM describes the liver's function as smoothing and regulating the flow of vital energy and blood, thus helping the free flow of Qi through the whole body. It also helps the spleen to send nutrient essence up and the stomach to send food down, normalising digestion.

The Liver Channel (Yin) originates from the big toe, around the ankle and rises up the inside of the leg into the body past the hip and finishing at the lower rib area. The Gall Bladder Channel (Yang) originates from an area at the outer corner of the eye, runs around the ear, over the side of the head, down the neck to the shoulder, underneath the shoulder and down the side of the body past the hip, descending down the outside of the leg to the ankle, then along the outside of the foot and finishing on the outside of the fourth toe.

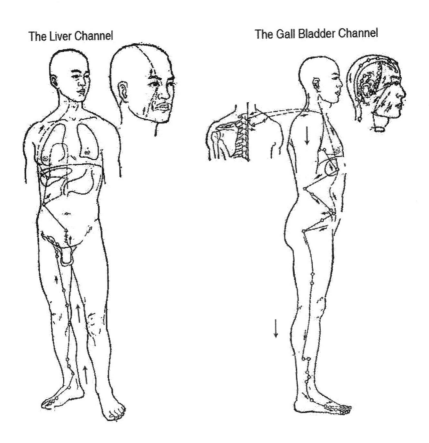

The Liver Channel

The Gall Bladder Channel

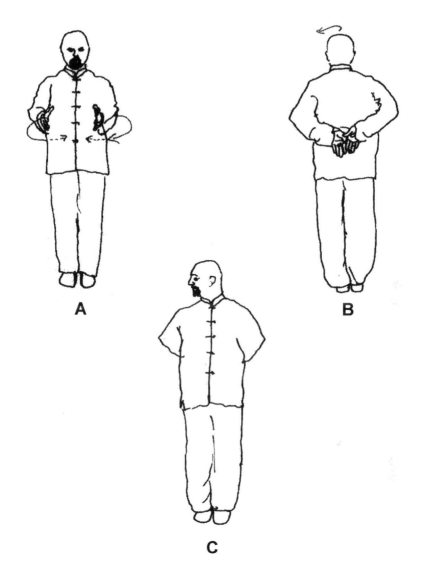

A Stand with feet together, toes gently gripping the ground, eyes focused in front (stimulating the Liver Channel).

B With palms facing outwards and fingers pointing downward, support your back by placing the back of your hands on your back over the kidneys.

C Let the breath out and on the next in-breath, turn your head to your left, looking over the left shoulder and gently twisting the spine (stimulating the Gall Bladder Channel). Breathe out as you turn back to the front.

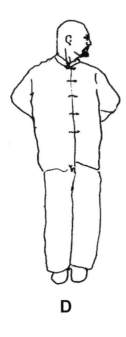
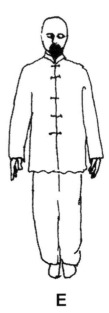

D   **E**

D Breathing in from centre position, turn to the right. Let your eyes draw a line around the room or sweep across the horizon. Check that the shoulders are facing straight ahead and that you are turning only the head and neck. Try to look around a bit more each time.

Repeat 4 times to each side.

E Return to basic stance – stand, arms at the sides, feet together and close the eyes. Relax and feel.

Fifth Piece – Stimulating and strengthening the whole body

This section is also good for memory and concentration. It's important not to have aggression when punching; keep the jaw relaxed, concentrate and focus.

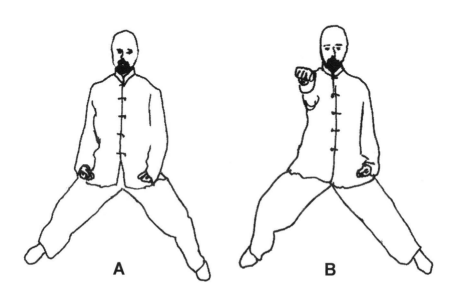

A Standing in wider horse-riding stance, use toes to grip the earth strongly. Grip the fists, keeping the thumb on the outside over the middle finger, holding strongly like a tiger's claw. Tense the whole body (about 40% - 50%). Rest both fists on the thighs, palms facing upwards.

B Breathe in and on the next out-breath extend the left fist out to the front of the body, turning the palm over to face the ground.

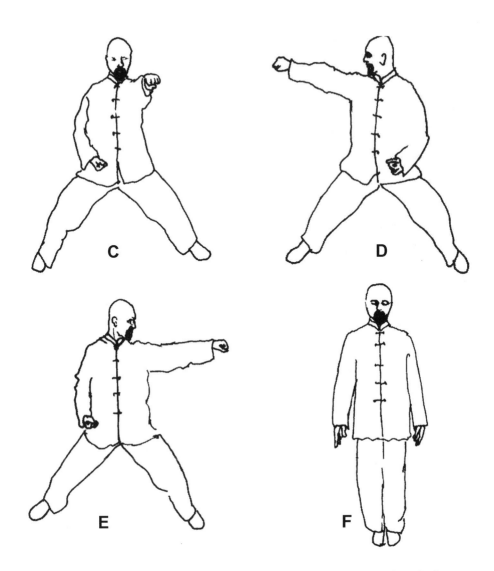

C Breathe in and bring your fist back onto the thigh, palm facing up. Repeat with the right hand.

D On the next movement, extend left fist to the side of the body, level with the shoulder. Let your eyes follow your hand.

E Then repeat to the right side. Without moving aggressively, focus your attention as you extend the energy to the horizon.

Repeat 4 times to each side.

F Return to basic stance – stand, arms at the sides, feet together and close the eyes. Relax and feel.

Sixth Piece – Regulating the Kidney and Bladder Channels

The kidneys regulate water circulation in the body and help maintain fluid balance. In TCM, the kidneys store the essence received from food and air and release it when required by the other organs. Thus, they are like the batteries of the body. Essence is also received from our parents and stored in the kidneys. The kidneys transform the essence into Qi or energy. They are very important organs and it's important to keep the kidneys and their water warm.

The Kidney Channel (Yin) originates from the sole of the foot, Yongquan, and rises up around the inside of the ankle, the inside of the leg, and through the abdomen to the chest below the collar bone. The Bladder Channel (Yang) originates from an area near the eyebrow, just off centre, goes back over the head descending down the back to the hip area, continues down the outside of the legs to the heel, along the outside of the foot, finishing on the outside of the small toe.

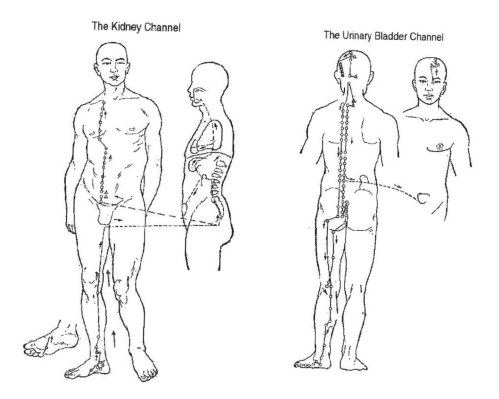

The Kidney Channel

The Urinary Bladder Channel

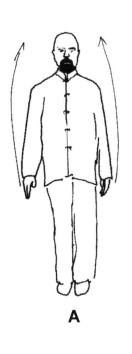

A

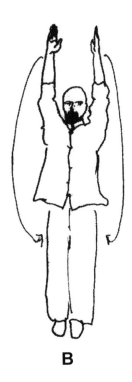

B

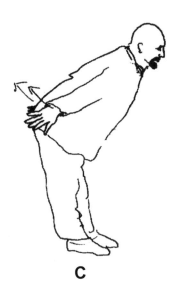

C

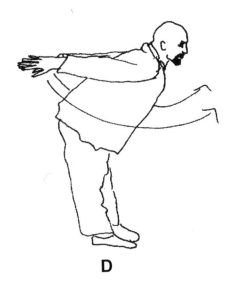

D

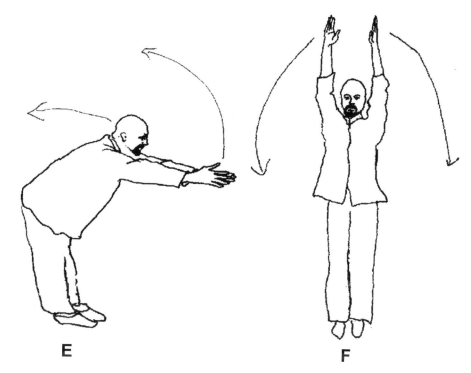

E   **F**

A   Standing with feet together, bring the arms up overhead. The palms face each other about shoulder width apart, as if holding a ball.

B, C Keeping the knees, back and elbows straight, bend at the hips and push the bottom back. As you rock back on your heels, toes gently gripping the ground, let the arms swing straight and parallel to each other, back behind the hips.

D, E, Breathe out, bring the arms down in front of body and pull the head
F   back to look at the horizon. Breathe in, push from the legs and swing arms up overhead. Look straight ahead and keep the back, elbows and knees straight (stimulating the Kidney and Bladder Channels). Swing like a pendulum.

Repeat 8 times.

Return to basic stance – stand, arms at the sides, feet together and close the eyes. Relax and feel.

Seventh Piece – Regulating the Heart, Small Intestine and Pericardium Channels

The heart is the Emperor of the body according to the ancient TCM texts. It propels the blood through the blood vessels and circulates it through the body. It is also where the spirit resides. If the Emperor is in good spirits, harmony prevails throughout the whole kingdom, the body and the universe.

The Heart Channel (Yin) originates from the centre of the armpit to the bicep, past the elbow to the outside of the wrist finishing at the end of the small finger. The Pericardium Channel (Yin), which also relates to the heart channel, starts next to the nipple and also flows down the centre of the inside of the arm, finishing at the middle finger. The Small Intestine Channel (Yang) starts from the outside tip of the little finger and runs upward along the outside of the arm through the wrist and elbow to the shoulder, then to the neck and cheek and finishes near the ear, at the depression where the mouth is opened.

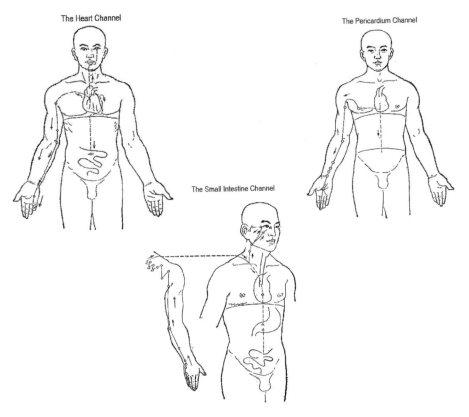

The Heart Channel

The Pericardium Channel

The Small Intestine Channel

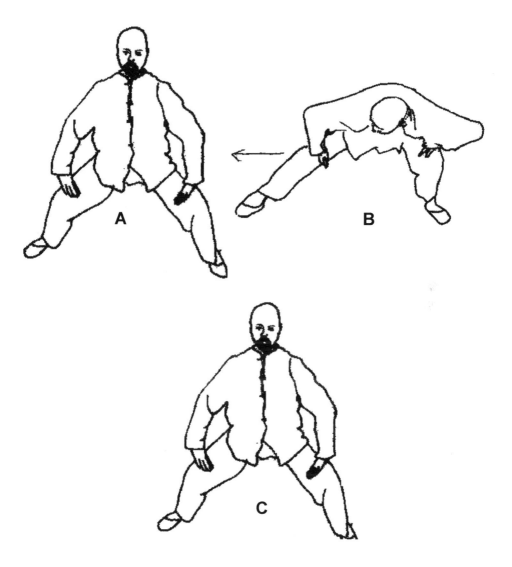

A Standing in the wider horse-riding stance, open tiger's mouth on both hands, keeping fingers together and flat. Place hands on the thighs, fingers pointing toward the inside, thumbs on outside of thighs.

B Breathe in, push the hips and bottom back, shift your weight over the right knee and turn your head to the left, looking up toward the sky. Push down on the outside of the right small finger to stimulate the Heart Channel and Small Intestine Channel.

C Breathe out, move back to centre, pulling the bottom in, looking to the front.

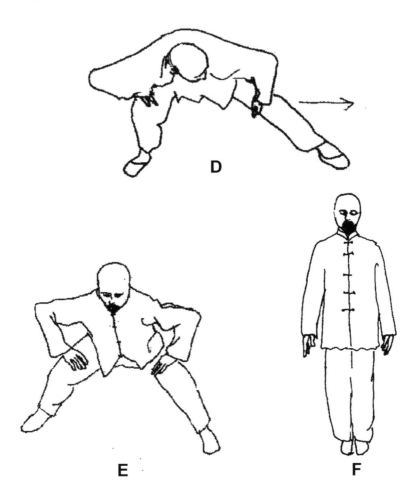

D

E

F

D Repeat on the other side: push hips back, shift your weight over the left knee and look up to the right. Push down on the outside of the left small finger to stimulate the Heart Channel and Small Intestine Channel. Keep the back straight, but don't straighten the legs. Keep knees off lock and don't let the head go below the heart.

E Breathe out, move back to centre, pulling the bottom in, looking to the front.

Repeat 4 times to each side.

F Return to basic stance – stand, arms at the sides, feet together and close the eyes. Relax and feel.

Eighth Piece – Spinal Jolt

This final section stimulates the energy up the back and to all the organs.

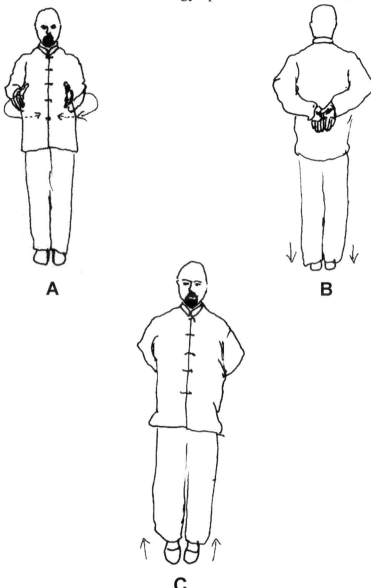

A

B

C

A, B Standing with feet together, place back of hands on your back, palms out as in the Fourth Piece, supporting the back. Let the breath out.

C On the next in-breath, go up onto the toes.

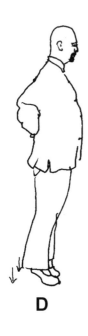

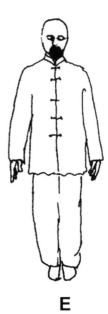

D

D   On the out-breath let the body drop onto the heels with a jolting action. Feel your way, trying it gently at first. Don't hurt yourself.

Repeat 8 times.

E   Return to basic stance – stand, arms at the sides, feet together and close the eyes. Relax and feel.

Close with meditation

The final stage is meditation, either cross-legged on the floor or on the edge of a chair keeping the back straight. The chin is tucked in, with the tip of the tongue on the top palate of the mouth, just behind the teeth. Breathe naturally in and out through the nose, sensing the breath and sensing the peace. Allow the breath to become smooth and even and the mind to rest (five minutes). Turn the hands in over the Dan Tian, the area beneath the navel, with one hand on top of the other. Allow your mind, breath and energy to settle. When breathing in, the abdomen gently pushes out into your hands and when breathing out gently push the hands in. Relax and feel the whole body breathe (five minutes). After the face rubbing practice (next chapter) place the hands palm down on the knees sensing the peace, the inner peace. Through the peace allow the heart to open like a smile, a wave of loving kindness permeating from the heart through the whole body. Just relax and let it go out through every cell. Every cell of the body is smiling with the radiance of the universe as you become one with the universe (five minutes).

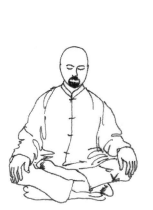
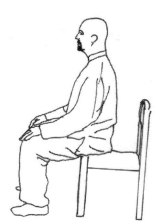

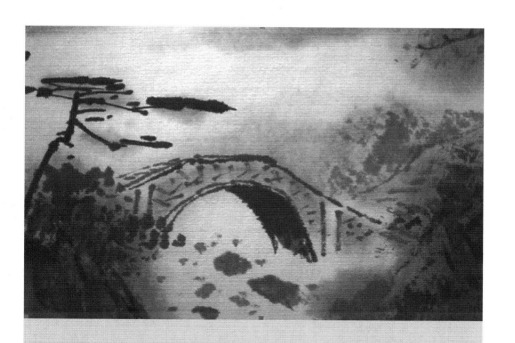

Chapter 8

Gathering the Qi
and Rubbing the Face

The Art of Life

Gathering the Qi and Rubbing the Face

The practice of Qigong helps clear the energy channels and dredges the meridians of stagnant Qi. This allows the Qi to flow smoothly through the body and creates an energy or Qi field.

We generally feel this Qi field in the hands. To gather and refine the Qi move the hands in and out as follows:

Gathering the Qi

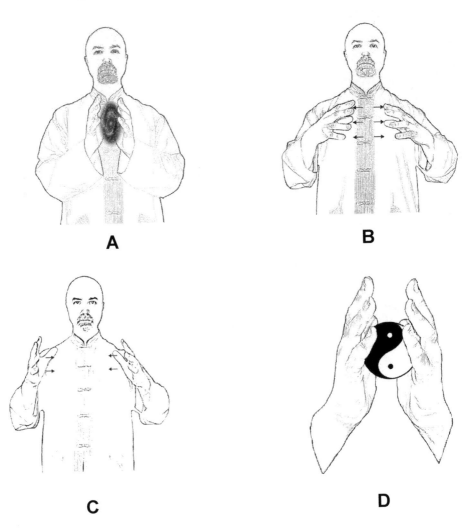

A

B

C

D

A Hold the hands in front of the body at chest height as if holding a ball of energy or light.

B Slightly draw the hands away from each other tensing the fingers.

C Then push the hands closer compressing the Qi between the hands.

Repeat six times.

D Relax and feel. We will generally feel warmth, like a field of energy between the hands. This creates a polarity as the left hand is Yang (positive) and the right hand is Yin (negative).

Now that the hands are charged with Qi it's a time for healing by placing the hands on a sore or injured part of your body or by massaging the face. Your face has many meridian acupuncture points that connect the meridians to the internal organs.

Face rubbing

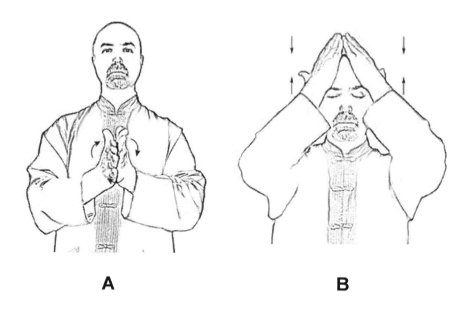

A   **B**

A   Rub the hands together and bring the healing energy through your heart into your hands.

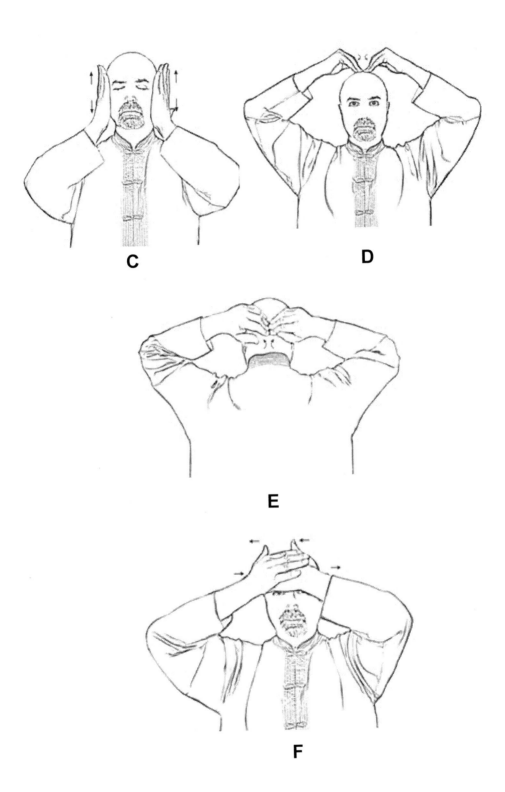

C

D

E

F

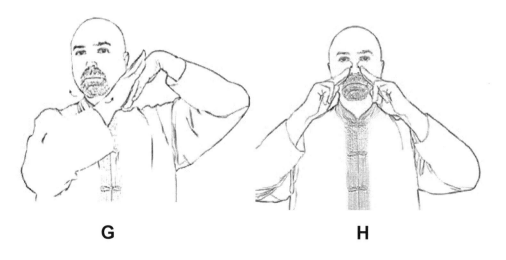

G
H

B, C Place the warm palms over your eyes (liver). Feel the warmth going in. Then rub the hands up and down from the forehead to the chin, the side of the face, then around the eyes and cheeks in a circular motion, like washing the face.

Rub around the ears with the tip of the fingers massaging around the outside of the ears down to the ear lobe. With the tips of the fingers, massage around the inside of the ear following all the grooves, stimulating the kidneys.

D, E With the tips of the fingers, massage back through the hair and then rub the back of the neck. Gently massage the base of the skull, the top of the head and massage up over the head and scalp.

F, G, H With one hand on top of the other rub the palm across the forehead and then rub around the chin letting the knuckles massage the jaw. Rub the fingers down the sides of the nose and around the cheek bones (lung).

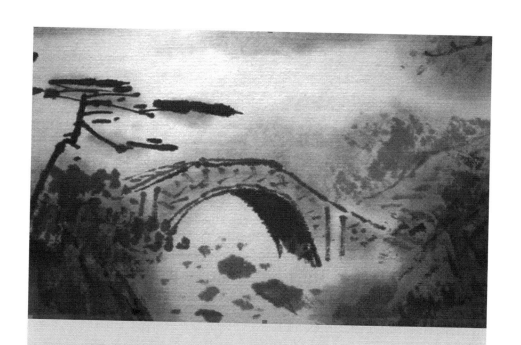

Chapter 9

Tai Ji Qigong Shibashi

太極氣功十八式

The Art of Life

Taiji Qigong Shibashi

Taiji (Tai Chi) is a Chinese term describing the Yin/Yang symbol. This symbol comprises two opposing forces that balance or complement each other. Without one the other would not exist. Yang energy is expressed in qualities such as up, external, male, hot and bright. Yin energy resides in the opposing characteristics; down, internal, female, cold and dark. When we find balance, we understand and achieve Tai Chi.

The popular soft, internal martial art called Taijiquan (Tai Chi Chuan) is a relatively new style and has been developed over the last 600 years. A verbal translation of 'Taijiquan' would be 'the interaction of Yin/Yang (Taiji) in creating the fist or boxing (Quan)'. There are many physical, emotional and energetic benefits to gain from practising Taijiquan forms, as well as self-defence applications.

Qigong is the ancient Chinese art of longevity. It is one of the components of the holistic system of Traditional Chinese Medicine, developed over 6,000 years. 'Qi' (Chi) is the energy of life, the vital energy that flows through the network of meridians in the body and connects with the energy of the universe. 'Gong' is a term which translates to work, mastery and training. Literally, Qigong is a way of working with the energy of life.

Shibashi translates to 'eighteen forms'. It is a newer set of movements that was developed in 1980 by Tai Chi Chuan Master He Weiqi and Qigong Master Lin Hou Sheng in Shanghai, China. It utilises Yang style Tai Chi Chuan postures and ancient Qigong movements. Combined with Traditional Chinese Medicine theory, it's a very powerful and complete system of Qigong. The interaction of Yin and Yang help bring harmony to the mind, body and breath.

What is the difference between Taiji (Tai Chi) and Qigong?

Qigong is a general term used since the early 1900s that describes all the Chinese energy techniques. There are three main categories Martial, Medical and Spiritual. Tai Chi Chuan can be described as a martial form of Qigong. But a good way to differentiate between the two is to contrast the ways in which they are practised. Practising Tai Chi Chuan is similar to shadow boxing with an imaginary opponent – blocking, striking, using the opponent's energy with yours to find balance (Tai Chi) – whereas Qigong movements are practised purely to cultivate one's own Qi, allowing it to connect with the Qi or energy of the universe.

Benefits of Tai Chi Qigong Shibashi

There are many long-term benefits from regular practice of Tai Chi Qigong Shibashi. It helps on the physical level by stimulating the blood circulation and exercising all the major joints, tendons, and muscles, and it increases flexibility and muscle tone. It also massages all the major internal organs. On an energetic level, it helps strengthen the Qi (vital energy) and stimulate the meridian system, which calms the mind and body, and reduces stress. This enables the mind to become clear and lets the heart open, creating a state of positive wellbeing and bringing harmony with the universe.

Main points

Movements should be slow, soft and smooth. Keep the same rhythm without pauses or speeding up. The body is upright with the back straight; relax all joints and muscles. Imagine that you are swimming in a crystal clear lake. Breathe in and out through the nose at all times. Some movements are longer than others. Coordinate your breath with the movement. Importantly, don't force any movement and don't force the breath. Make it a natural and enjoyable experience. Each movement is practised 6 times equalling 108 movements or 108 breaths.

Please note that the images are mirrored for the reader; just follow in the same direction.

Basic stance

Stand with feet parallel, shoulder-width apart, as if standing on train tracks, with knees slightly off lock. Let your weight sink into your legs, feet and into the ground. Keep the coccyx or tail bone slightly tucked in, chest relaxed, and the back straight. Hold your arms away from the body, fingers open and relaxed pointing to the earth, palms facing the body. With the chin slightly tucked in and the top of the head (Bai Hui point) reaching to the sky as if a silken cord attached to it is lifting the whole body, light the Hui Yin, gently squeezing the pelvic floor. Relax your eyes and face and look out into the distance. Keeping your jaw relaxed, place the tip of the tongue on the top palate of your mouth, just behind the front teeth. Breathe in and out through the nose. When breathing in, let the abdomen push out slightly and as the breath comes out, let the abdomen contract. Just relax, letting the whole body breathe.

(See next page for diagrams)

Basic Stance Cont'd.

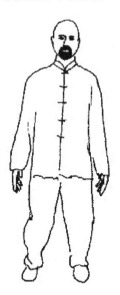 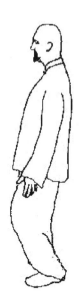

Movement No. 1 – Raising arms

Benefit – Awakens the Qi, activates the meridian system, stimulates the kidneys regulates the blood circulation, balances blood pressure, and helps calm the nerves. The gentle movements of the arms and legs smooth the energy channels and help prevent arthritis.

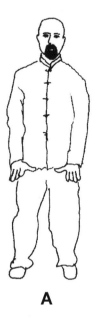 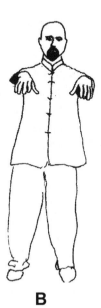

A   B

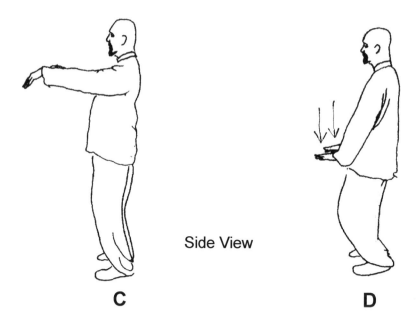

Side View

C   D

A   Push your legs into the ground, gripping slightly with the toes, and breathe in.

B, C   Feel the momentum rise up the spine as you lift your arms to shoulder height. Shoulders, elbows and wrists are relaxed with the fingers pointing to ground, over the knees.

D   Breathe out, move your weight back on your heels, fingers flick out gently, like small ripples going out across the clear lake. Then lower arms as you bend your legs and return to the basic stance.

Continue 6 times.

Movement No. 2 – Opening the chest (Heart)

Benefit – Helps with the function of the heart and lungs, increases breathing capacity, and increases Qi and blood circulation. It is also beneficial for people with depression, insomnia and hypertension.

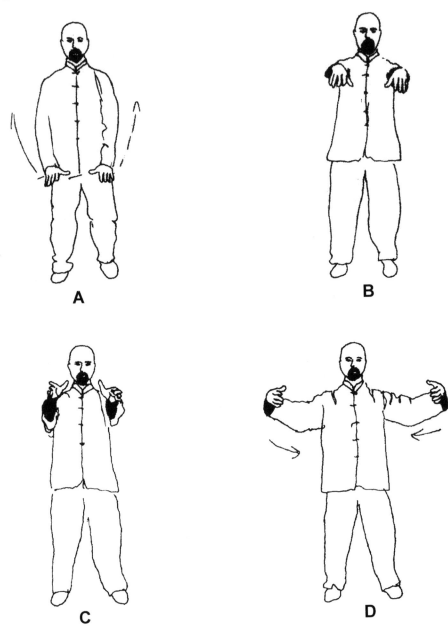

A

B

C

D

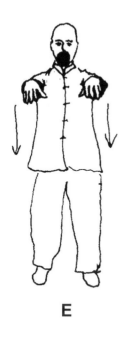

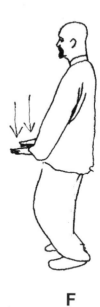

E   F

A   Push the legs into the ground as in movement No. 1, breathe in.

A, B, Bring the arms up and as they reach shoulder height, they open,
C   as if a large balloon is expanding from the chest. Draw open the arms
         and chest as if opening to the beautiful scene in front of you, while
         making sure the arms do not push back behind the body.

D   Breathe out and push arms in again as if squeezing the balloon.

E, F When they reach shoulder width, turn the palms to face the ground
         and lower your arms as you gently bend your knees back to the basic
         stance.

Continue 6 times.

Movement No. 3 – Painting the rainbow

Benefit – Helps regulate blood pressure as well as aiding digestion, relieving stomach aches and easing shoulder pain.

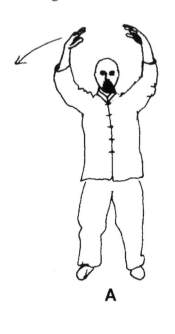

A

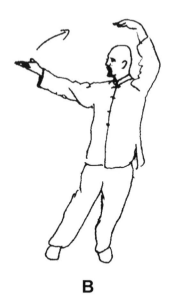

B

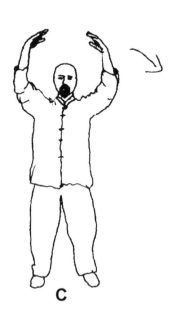

C

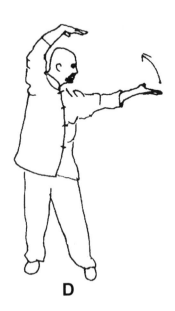

D

A Breathe in. Raise the arms over the head, like holding a big ball.

B Move your weight horizontally 60° onto your right leg. Breathe out, relax the left hip, the right palm faces top of head, the Bai Hui point. Let left arm move down to shoulder height with the palm facing up.

C, D Breathe in, push from right leg, moving weight 60°onto your left leg. Breathe out, relax right hip as the left palm faces top of head and looking at right palm which is facing the sky. Coordinate the arms and legs as you shift your weight from one leg to the other. Maintain momentum from feet to hands in one movement with no breaks. Imagine the hands are like a paint brush and you are painting a rainbow across the sky. <u>Important</u> – remain at the same level and do not bend your knees up and down.

Continue 3 to each side.

Movement No. 4 – Separating the clouds
Benefit – Helps stimulate kidneys, increase vital energy (original Qi), strengthens legs and waist.

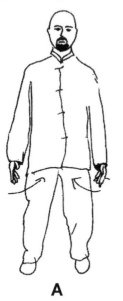

A

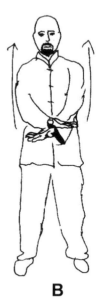

B

A From basic stance, breathe in while pushing down with the legs.

A, B With your hands in front, let them rise up in front of your face as if scooping up water.

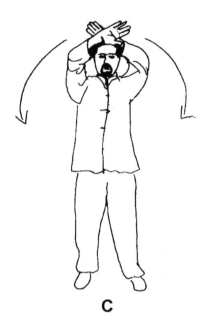

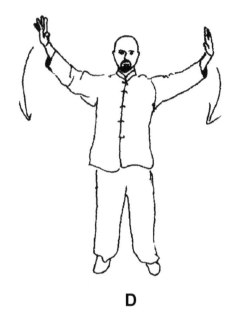

C   Rolling the shoulders and keeping them relaxed, separate the arms, palms facing out.

D   Breathe out, letting your arms continue down to shoulder height at the side of the body. Make sure arms don't move behind your body. Lower the knees together with the arms, like a parachutist, bracing your fall. Each time, imagine reaching into the sky, separating the clouds and letting the light shine down on you.

Continue 6 times.

Movement No. 5 – Rolling arms

Benefit – Good for shoulders, elbows, wrists and respiratory function. Also beneficial for people with neurasthenia, arthritis and asthma.

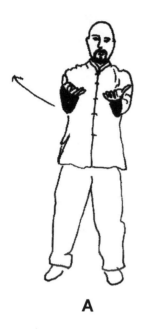

A

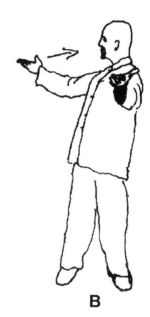

B

A Raise the arms in front of the body, palms facing up, as if holding a big ball.

B Breathe in as you draw the left elbow back to the waist, relax left hip as left arm sweeps 90° to the side, making sure to keep the right arm in front.

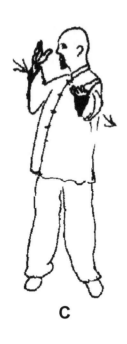

C

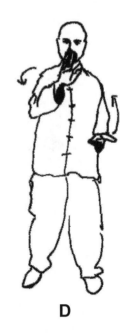

D

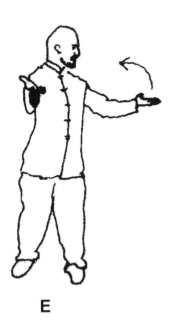

E

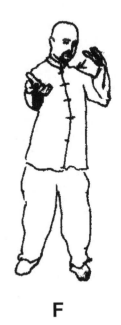

F

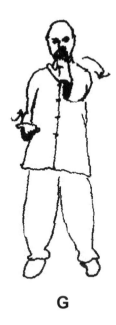

G

C Let the left hand rise to ear height, keeping the elbow down. Relax left wrist, letting the hand become limp.

D Breathe out, relax right hip and let the momentum move from the left hand as it pushes forward while the right arm draws back to the waist.

E Finish with the left hand in front of body, looking across the finger tips while the right elbow is at waist, palm facing the sky. Breathe in as right arm sweeps 90° to the side, left palm turns up to the sky, remaining in front of body.

F Let right hand rise to ear height, keeping the elbow down.

G Breathe out, relax the left hip, push the right hand as you let the left elbow pull back to the waist. Looking across the right finger tips; imagine pushing through the water and pushing a lotus flower off the palm of your hand.

Continue 3 to each side.

Movement No. 6 – Rowing boat in the middle of the lake

Benefit – Helps the digestive system, clears the head and calms the nerves. Beneficial for people with backache and headache.

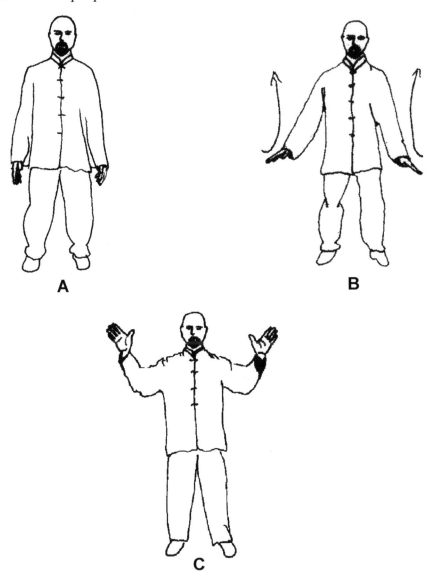

A

B

C

A, B, Breathe in, push from the legs and let arms rise to the side; think
C of the top of the head and tip of the thumbs.

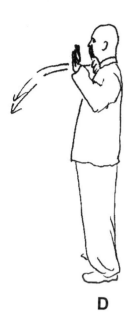

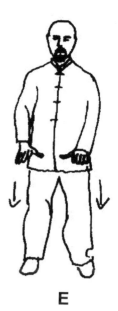

D

E

D, E When arms reach shoulder height, roll them over in front of body with palms facing the ground. Remember to keep the elbows down. Breathe out. In coordination with the legs, let the arms move down in front of body as in movement No 1. Imagine rowing a boat.

Continue 6 times.

Movement No. 7 – Supporting a ball in front of the shoulders

Benefit – Helps release physical and mental stress, relaxes the chest inducing deeper breathing. By focusing the eyes on the upward hand it is possible to induce a state of self-hypnosis, It is also beneficial for those suffering from insomnia and helps balance blood pressure.

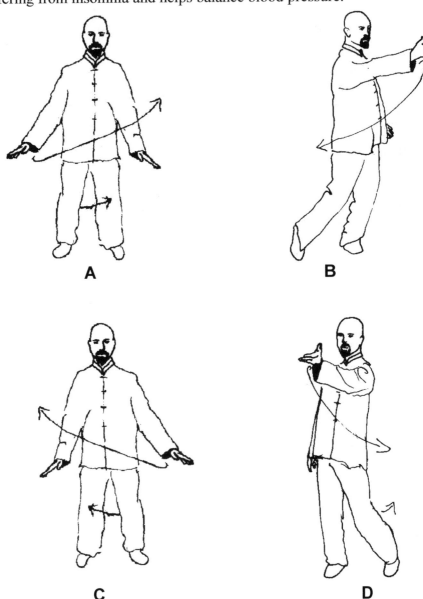

A

B

C

D

A Push down on the right leg as the left hand scoops up; move weight to the right leg as you lift the left heel.

B Relax right hip as the left arm rises to shoulder height, palm facing up, as if supporting a ball in front of your shoulder.

C Breathe out. Left palm turns over and sweeps down as your left heel is placed on the ground. Centre your weight, finishing in basic stance.

D For the other side, push down on the left leg as right hand scoops up, moving your weight to the left leg as you lift the right heel. Relax the left hip as the right arm rises to shoulder height, palm facing up. Breathe out, right palm turns over and sweeps down as your right heel is placed on the ground, centering your weight. Keep an even, steady pace, like the swing of a pendulum.

Continue 3 to each side.

Movement No. 8 – Gazing at the moon

Benefit – Helps strengthen the spleen, kidney and digestive system as well as helping back pain.

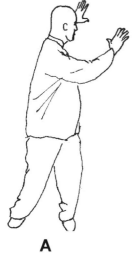
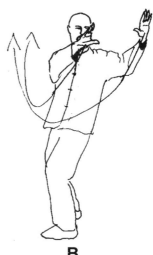

A   **B**

A With both feet firmly on the ground, breathe in. Swing both arms to your right 90° to about shoulder height. With palms facing out, look through window of your hands as if gazing up at the moon.

B Breathe out, relax the left arm. Let the palm face up and allow momentum to swing both arms down as if holding a balloon in your hands to the centre of the body.

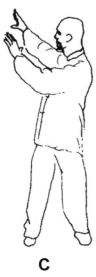

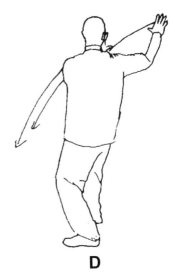

C   D

C Breathe in. Both arms continue to swing in a circular motion 90° to your left to about shoulder height, palms facing out, again as if gazing at the moon.

D Breathe out, relax right arm, palm faces up and momentum swings both arms down.

Continue 3 to each side.

Movement No. 9 – Turning waist and pushing the wind

Benefit – Helps strengthen the spleen and kidney, promotes leg and back energy and helps back pain.

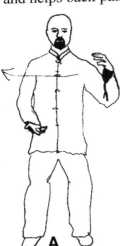

A   B

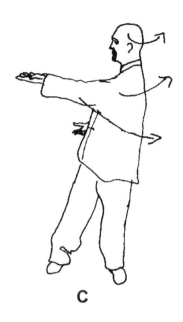

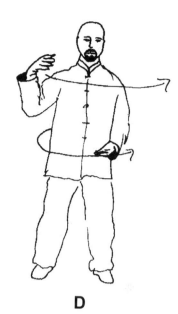

C   D

A From the previous movement, gazing at the moon to your left, breathe in. Let both arms swing down, the left elbow draws into the left waist, palm facing up on the left hip, as your right hand swings up to your right ear, keeping the elbow down. Look at right hand.

B Breathe out, relax left hip, turn waist pushing right palm 90° to your left. <u>Importantly</u>, keep the elbow relaxed - don't push all the way.

C Breathe in, relax right hand as the palm turns up to the sky.

D Turn from waist, drawing back the right elbow 90° to face the front. Let the left hand swing up to left ear, keeping the elbow down. Again, look at the left hand.

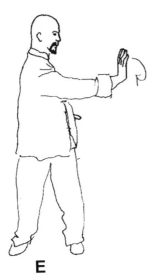

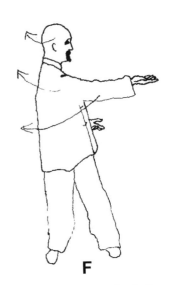

E

F

E Breathe out, relax the right hip and turn the waist, pushing the left palm 90° to your right. Remember, not all the way.

F Breathe in. Relax the left hand as the palm turns up to the sky. Turn from the waist, drawing back the left elbow 90° to face the front. Imagine pushing your palm through water and watching the waves ripple out to the distance.

Continue 3 to each side.

Movement No. 10 – Moving the hands in the clouds

Benefit – Helps stimulate Qi and blood circulation as well as the digestive system. Helps prevent arthritis.

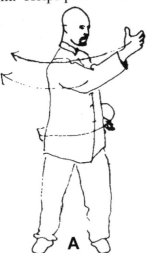

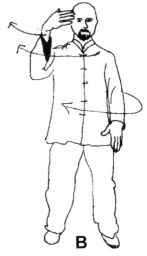

A

B

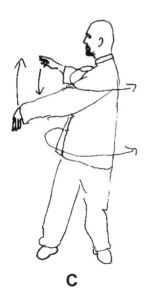

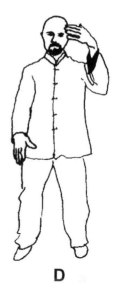

C   **D**

A   From the previous movement, push the left palm to your right. Breathe in. Relax the left hand, turning the palm towards the face as if looking into a mirror; the Lao Gong point faces the Upper Dan Tian, whilst the right palm turns towards the navel (abdomen), and the Lao Gong point faces the Dan Tian.

B, C From the waist, turn the whole body to your left about 180° or as far as feels comfortable. Breathe out, reversing the position of the hands. The right hand swings up, palm in front of the face; as the left hand swings down, palm moves towards the navel. Remember to do this movement slowly.

D   Breathe in and turn the whole body from the waist to your right about 180° or as far as feels comfortable. Imagine standing on a mountain moving your hands in the clouds.

Continue 3 to each side.

Movement No. 11 – Scooping the sea and looking at the sky

Benefit – Helps strengthen the thigh and waist muscles, improves blood circulation, balances blood pressure and massages the internal organs.

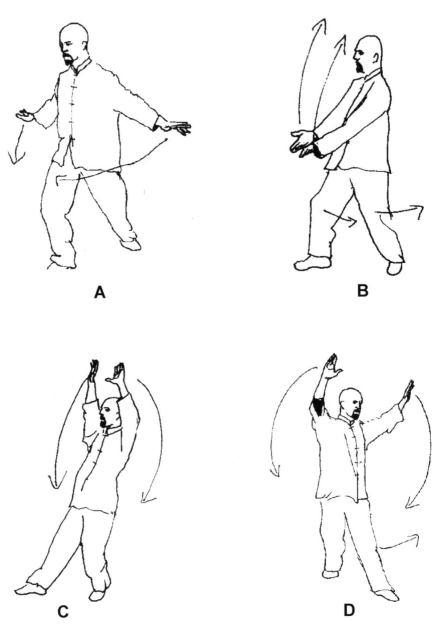

A

B

C

D

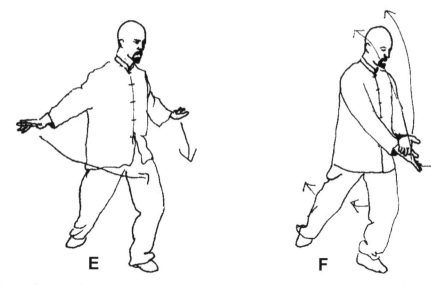

E   F

From the previous movement, bring both arms to the front and to the basic stance.

A   Breathe in, raising left leg as you raise both arms and step forward 45° to your left. Breathe out, push from the right (back) leg moving the weight forward, about 60° over the left foot.

B   Hands scoop up, crossed at the wrists as if scooping up water. Eyes are looking 45° down at the sea.

C   Breathe in, push from the left (front) leg, moving about 60% of your weight back, keeping left toe on the ground. The arms move back with the body, in front of the face. Relax the shoulders and separate the hands as you look 45° up to the sky. The arms continue in a circle past the shoulders – the arms do not go behind body. Breathe out, push from the back leg forward, keeping momentum to scoop up the sea.

Continue 3 times.

D   After third repetition, when pushing back with left leg, bring the feet back together while looking at the sky. Simultaneously, step right leg forward 45° to the right as arms pass the shoulder.

E, F Breathe out, push from the left (back) leg to scoop the sea another 3 times.

Important – keep the back heel on the ground and don't move all your weight to the front when pushing forward.

Movement No. 12 – Pushing the waves

Benefit – Helps strengthen the liver and spleen as well as your legs and waist. It is beneficial for those with hypertension.

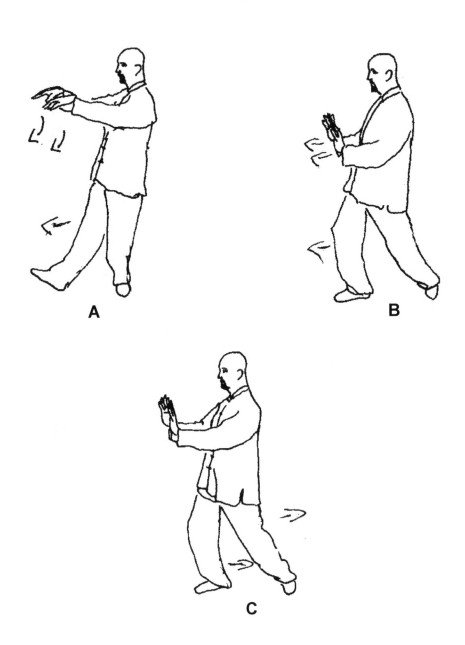

A   B

C

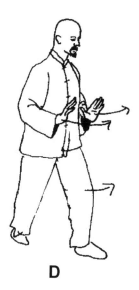 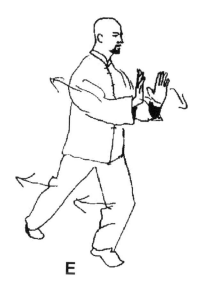

| D | E |

From the previous movement, bring the feet back together.

A   As in movement No. 11, raise the left leg, breathing in, and step forward 45° to your left. Raise the arms in front of the body as in movement No. 1.

B   Breathe out, move the arms down to waist height, relax the wrists, palms facing forward and push from the right (back) leg, moving 60% of your weight forward. <u>Important,</u> do not extend the elbows, but keep the arms relaxed. Breathe in and relax the wrists with the fingers facing the ground.

C   Push back from the left (front) leg letting the toe come off the ground. The arms move back with the body. Do not bend the elbow; keep it in a fixed position.

Continue 3 times. Imagine pushing and riding the waves.

D, E   After the third repetition, when pushing back with the left leg, bring the feet back together and keep the arms in front. Step forward 45° to the right and push the waves 3 times. Again, keep the back heel on the ground when pushing forward.

Movement No. 13 – Flying dove spreads its wings

Benefit – Helps strengthen the liver and spleen as well as increasing lung capacity and helping the digestive system.

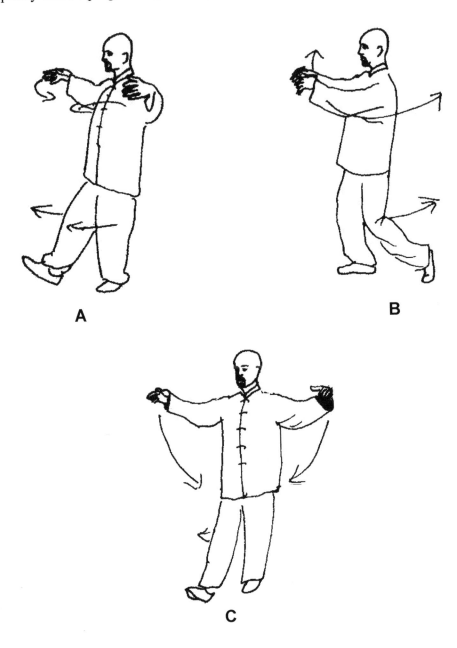

A

B

C

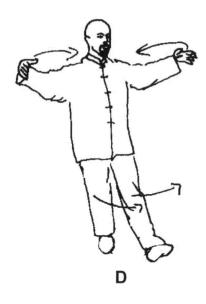

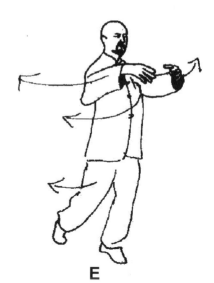

D
E

A   From the previous movement, with the feet together, raise the left leg, and on the in breath, again step forward 45° to your left as both arms rise to the side.

B   Breathe out, push from the back leg, moving weight 100% forward which brings the right (back) heel off the ground, balancing on the front leg. Let both arms form a circle in front of the chest like holding a big balloon.

C   Breathe in and push from the front leg to the back as arms expand, opening the chest as in movement No 2. Maintain the momentum from feet to hands. Imagine a bird in flight, spreading the Qi through the whole body.

Continue 3 times.

D, E After the third repetition, bring the feet back together keeping the arms to your side. Step forward 45° to your right and spread your wings another 3 times.

Movement No. 14 – Punching in basic stance

Benefit – Helps increase lung capacity, and strengthens the whole body.

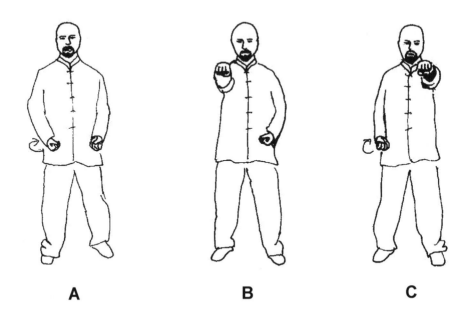

A   **B**   **C**

A After the previous movement, breathe in and hold the fists as if holding a small egg in your hands. Don't clench your fists. Both fists sit on thighs, palms facing up. Open the chest a little.

B As you breathe out, the left fist spirals out in front of the left shoulder, palm facing ground. Keep your elbow off lock, and relax.

C Breathe in. Draw left fist in to the waist. Breathe out as the right fist spirals out in front of the right shoulder. Look to the distance. Imagine the breath and energy extending out to the distance.

Continue 3 to each side.

Movement No. 15 – The flying wild goose

Benefit – Helps strengthen the spleen and kidney, relieves inner tensions and has a liberating effect on the body and spirit. Improves and balances blood pressure.

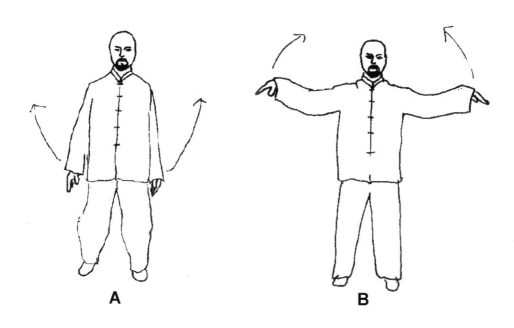

A   **B**

A After the previous movement, the arms come to the side in the basic stance. Breathe in, push the legs into the ground as in movement No. 1. Let the arms rise to the side to shoulder height, fingers and elbows pointing to the ground.

B Bring the heels off the ground as hands move towards the head, palms facing out, elbows down.

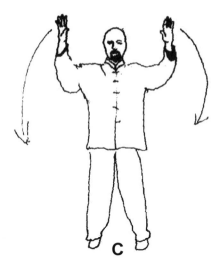

C Breathe out, let the heels come down onto the ground. The hands move down to shoulder height, palms facing down. Knees bend as arms come down to the side of the body in the basic stance. Imagine a bird in flight.

Continue 6 times.

Movement No. 16 – Rotating flywheel

Benefit – Massages the internal organs, strengthens the spirit and awakens the joy of life. Helps in the recovery of a tired body and reduces stiffness in the back.

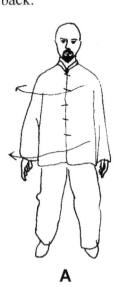

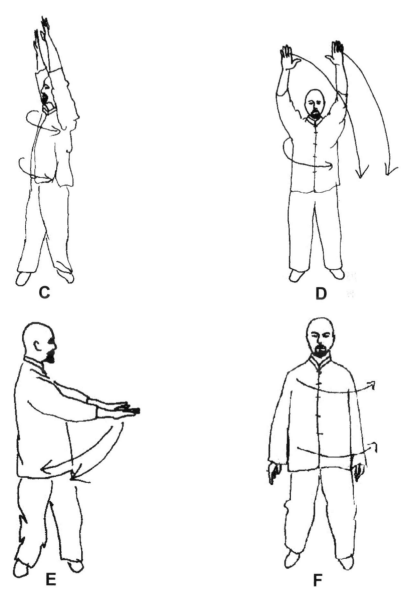

C

D

E

F

A   Turn the waist to your left.

B   Breathe in, push from legs, both arms rise up over the head.

C   Turn from the waist and let the arms follow the body about 180°
        to your right, keeping elbows and shoulders relaxed.

D, E,   Breathe out. The arms swing down as they pass your shoulders.
F, G   The knees sink in coordination. Move from the waist to your left
        in a big circle, turning the palms out.

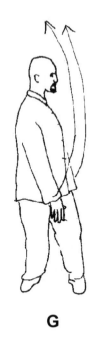

G

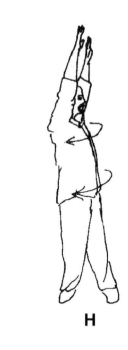

H

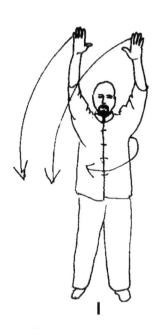

I

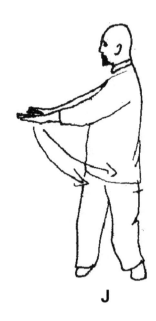

J

H, I, J After the third rotation, stop at the bottom and go back in the opposite direction. Move slowly in time with your breathing. Imagine turning a big wheel and mixing and absorbing the Qi from the sky (Yang) and the earth (Yin).

Return to basic stance.

Continue 6 times.

Movement No. 17 – Stepping and bouncing the ball

Benefit – Helps stimulate the meridian system, harmonises body movement and brings about a feeling of joy.

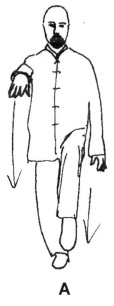

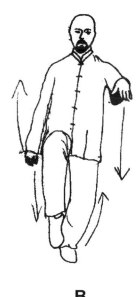

A | **B**

A Move your weight to your left. Breathe in. Let your left wrist rise at the same time as your right knee, balancing on one leg. Breathe out, let your left wrist go down with your right knee, placing toe first, then the heel.

B Move the weight to your right leg. Breathe in and let your right wrist rise at the same time as your left knee, again balancing on one leg. Breathe out. Let your right wrist go down with your left knee down, placing toe first, then heel. Imagine stepping and bouncing a ball.

Continue 3 times.

Movement No.18 – Balancing the Qi

Benefit – Regulates breathing and blood pressure, strengthens the kidneys and produces inner peace and calmness.

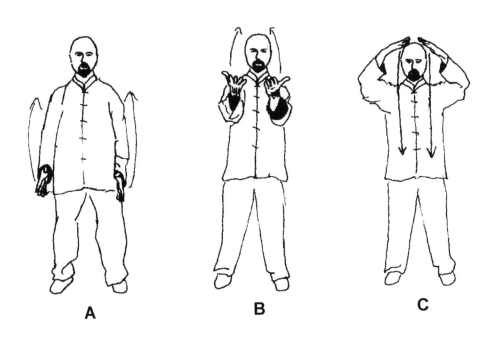

A   B   C

A Push the legs into the ground and, gripping the toes slightly, breathe in.

B Scoop hands to side and up in front of body. As momentum rises up the spine, straighten the legs slightly. Lift the arms to forehead height, keeping the elbows down.

C Turn the palms in to the top of the head and towards the ground. Breathing out, let the arms descend down the front of body. Put your weight back on the heels, lowering the arms in coordination with the legs. Balancing the Qi up the back (Yang) and down the front (Yin)

Continue 6 times.

Closing

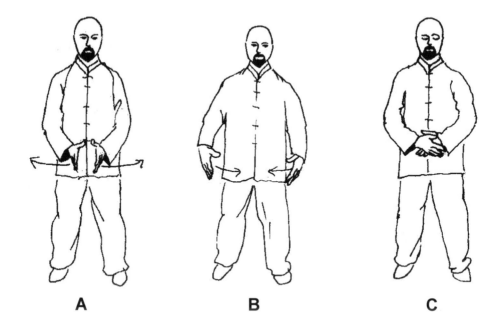

A   After the sixth balancing the Qi movement, the palms face each other like holding a small balloon or a ball of light in front of the abdomen. Breathe in, letting the balloon expand into your hands, pushing them apart, to about body width.

B, C Breathe out, gently squeeze the balloon bringing one palm over the other, connecting Lao Gong points in the palms of the hands and place both palms over the abdomen, the Dan Tian. Close your eyes allowing the breath, mind and energy to settle. As you breathe in, feel the abdomen gently push out into your hands. As you breathe out, gently push your hands in toward the abdomen. Relax, feel your whole body breathe. Stand like this for as long as feels comfortable or for at least six breaths.

To finish – Gathering the Qi and rubbing the face
(see Chapter 8 for diagrams)

When we have finished, rub the hands together. Feeling the warmth in your hands, place the warm, healing palms over your eyes. Feel the warmth going into the face, then rub the hands up and down from the forehead to the chin, the side of the face, then around the eyes and cheeks in a circular motion, like washing the face.

Rub around the ears with the tip of the fingers massaging around the outside of the ears down to the ear lobe. With the tips of the fingers, massage around the inside of the ear following all the grooves, stimulating the blood and Qi.

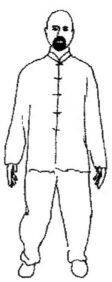

With the tips of the fingers, massage back through the hair, and then rub the back of the neck. Massage up over the head and scalp and with one hand on top of the other rub the palm across the forehead and then rub around the chin letting the knuckles massage the jaw. Rub the fingers down the sides of the nose and around the cheek bones.

Stand with arms at the side, feet together and close the eyes. Relax and feel.

Close with meditation

The final stage is meditation, either cross-legged on the floor or on the edge of a chair keeping the back straight. The chin is tucked in, with the tip of the tongue on the top palate of the mouth, just behind the teeth. Breathe naturally in and out through the nose. Relax and feel.

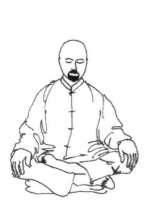 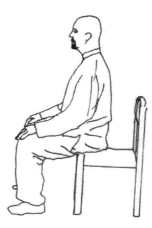

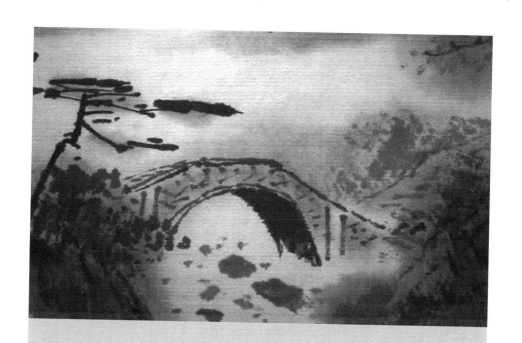

Chapter 10

The Five Element Qigong Meditation

The Art of Life

The Five Element Qigong Meditation

The Five Element Theory is an ancient understanding of the natural world. It's expressed and experienced through the consistent movement and transformation of our environment, and the elements are interrelated and influence each other. We as human beings are also an integral part of this system. This theory together with Yin and Yang are the main methods used in Traditional Chinese Medicine and Taoism to help explain our connection to and relationship with our environment and the universe.

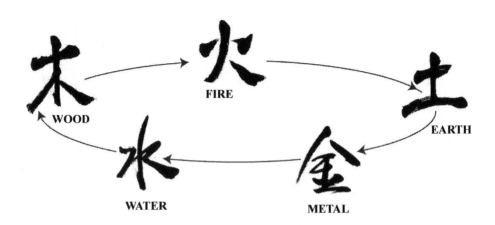

	HOU: FIRE	TU: EARTH	JIN: METAL	SHUI: WATER	MU: WOOD
Organ	Heart	Spleen	Lungs	Kidneys	Liver
Season	Summer	Late summer	Autumn	Winter	Spring
Emotion	Joy/excitement	Worry	Grief	Fear	Anger
Colour	Red	Yellow	White	Deep blue	Green

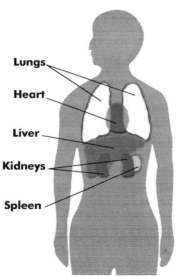

Lungs
Heart
Liver
Kidneys
Spleen

The Five Element Qigong Meditation focuses on the five solid (Yin) organs of the body and their corresponding element: Heart (Fire), Spleen (Earth), Lungs (Metal), Kidneys (Water) and Liver (Wood). These organs function a bit like batteries and when we bring our awareness and energy to them, they help our Qi flow smoothly and bring harmony to mind, body and spirit. The Qi from these organs then supplies the flowing (Yang) organs: Small Intestine (Fire), Stomach (Earth), Large Intestine (Metal), Urinary Bladder (Water) and Gall Bladder (Wood).

This meditation follows the progressive order of the Five Elements. The way to remember is to follow the natural order of nature, starting with the Heart relating to Summer, followed by the Spleen (late Summer), Lungs (Autumn), Kidneys (Winter) and Liver (Spring).

The Five Element Qigong Meditation follows this cycle three times. The first cycle is to become aware of the organ by sending our appreciation and gratitude, acknowledging the organ for the work that it does, and to consciously allow a coloured cloud to envelope the organ, dissolving the excess emotion. After clearing the stale energy, the next cycle energises the organ with our love and appreciation to become a precious stone, allowing the light from the universe to shine on the organ. The third cycle helps spread the Qi through the whole body with our love and smile, allowing all the organs to smile with the radiance of the universe.

Preparation Sit in a comfortable position either on a cushion or a chair, keeping the back straight. Gently breathing in and out through your nose, just relax, follow and watch the breath.

First cycle

After your mind has become calm and peaceful, place your awareness in the area of the **Heart**. With intention, send your appreciation and gratitude to the Heart, thanking it for the work that it does. The Heart represents the Element of Fire, the season of summer and its colour is a fiery red. The emotion of joy and excitement can affect the function of the Heart. With your intention, bring in a fiery red cloud from the universe and let it envelop the entire Heart, helping to dissolve the excess joy and excitement that may be stored there.

Now place your awareness in the area of the **Spleen**. This is next to the heart on the left hand side of the body, under the rib cage. With intention, send appreciation and gratitude to the Spleen. The Spleen represents the Element of Earth, the season of late summer and the colour is a golden/yellow. The emotion of worry can affect the function of the Spleen. With your intention, pull in a golden/yellow cloud from the universe and let it envelop the entire Spleen, helping to dissolve the excess worry which can be stored there.

Now place your awareness in the area of the **Lungs**. With intention send your appreciation and gratitude to the Lungs. The Lungs represent the Element of Metal, the season of Autumn and their colour is a silver/white. The emotion of grief can affect the function of the Lungs. With intention, draw in a silver/white cloud from the universe and let it envelop the entire lungs helping dissolve the excess grief which can be stored there.

Now place your awareness in the area of the **Kidneys**. With intention, send your appreciation and gratitude to the Kidneys. The Kidneys represent the Element of Water, the season of winter and the colour is a deep blue, like the colour of the deep ocean. The emotion of fear can affect the function of the Kidneys. With your intention, bring in a deep blue cloud from the universe and let it envelop the Kidneys in order to dissolve the excess fear which may be stored there.

Now place your awareness in the area of the **Liver**. With intention, send appreciation and gratitude to the Liver. The Liver represents the Element of Wood, the season of spring and the colour is a rich green, like the green of a new growth forest. The emotion of anger affects the function of the Liver. With your intention pull a rich green cloud in from the universe and let it envelop the entire Liver helping to dissolve the excess anger which can be stored there.

Second Cycle

With our love and appreciation, the **Heart** becomes a fiery red, precious stone, allowing the light from the universe to shine down on the heart, helping to open and heal the whole body. We can see it shining in the light. With our love and appreciation, the **Spleen** becomes a golden yellow precious stone, allowing the light from the universe to shine on the spleen. With our love and appreciation the **Lungs** become a silvery white precious stone, and with the light from the universe the chest opens. With our love and appreciation the **Kidneys** becomes a deep blue precious stone. With our love and appreciation, the **Liver** becomes a rich green precious stone and we can see it shining in the light. We open the chest, the treasure chest and let the light from the universe shine down on our whole body.

Third Cycle

With our love, smile and our loving kindness, we can see the **Heart** smiling as it appreciates the attention we are giving it. This helps open the energy channels of the body, connecting us with the universe. We see the smile spreading into the **Spleen**. The **Lungs** and the **Kidneys** are smiling, too, as well as the **Liver**, also smiling. Our whole beautiful body is smiling with the radiance of the universe, as we merge with the universe.

Closing

Rub the palms together. Consciously bring your healing energy, love and kindness through the heart into your hands. Place the palms over the heart, allowing the heart to absorb the warm healing energy. Then after a few minutes, place the palms over the spleen, followed by the lungs, kidney and liver. To finish the meditation, place one hand on top of the other over the lower Dan Tian, the energy centre just beneath the navel. Just relax and allow the breath and energy to settle.

Meditation Points

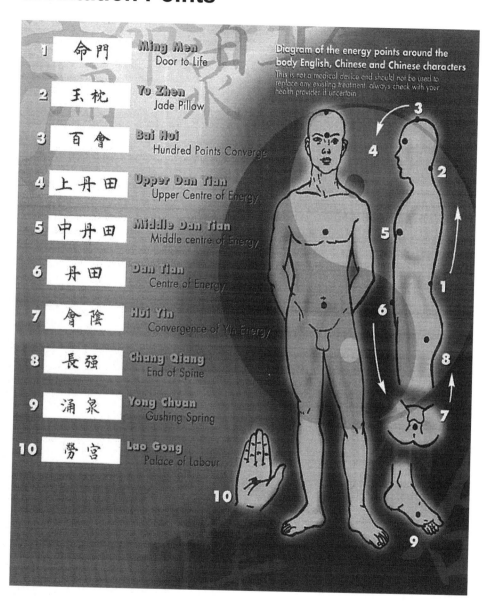

1	命門	**Ming Men**	Door to Life
2	玉枕	**Yu Zhen**	Jade Pillow
3	百會	**Bai Hui**	Hundred Points Converge
4	上丹田	**Upper Dan Tian**	Upper Centre of Energy
5	中丹田	**Middle Dan Tian**	Middle centre of Energy
6	丹田	**Dan Tian**	Centre of Energy
7	會陰	**Hui Yin**	Convergence of Yin Energy
8	長强	**Chang Qiang**	End of Spine
9	涌泉	**Yong Chuan**	Gushing Spring
10	勞宮	**Lao Gong**	Palace of Labour

Diagram of the energy points around the body English, Chinese and Chinese characters

This is not a medical device and should not be used to replace any existing treatment, always check with your health provider if uncertain

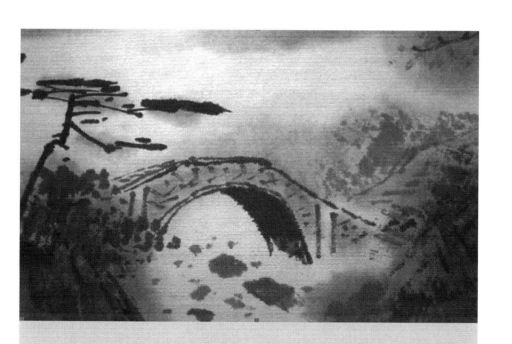

Chapter 11

Stories to Inspire

The Art of Life

Stories to inspire

I have been practising Qigong every day for sixteen years. Classes became available in my town and as a practicing yoga teacher I was looking for somewhere where I could be the student.

Qigong helps bring me right into the present moment with a feeling of immense serenity. Each year my health has improved and whenever I do experience a setback, gentle Qigong is always there to help me.

Over the years I have learnt to be more accepting of what life brings and learning the joy of peace. One of the lovely things about Qigong is the wonderful people it brings into my life. I have made some very special friends through the practice and would never have traveled to China if it had not been for Qigong. **Joan, Victoria**

I read a book about Qigong in 2005, but did not practise at that time. In 2006 I was diagnosed with cancer and then realised the importance of practising Qigong on a regular basis. I practised twice daily for six months, then daily for sometime. Currently, I only practise twice a week due to other work commitments.

Practising Qigong, particularly whilst in my healing process increased my Qi thus strengthening my body and preparing me for my journey of healing. Qigong also helped in calming my mind. I was able to think clearly which helped me to make rational decisions regarding my health.

When I practise Qigong now, I feel very relaxed and can feel different sensations throughout my body, particularly energy from my hands. The warm healing energy I feel after a session of Qigong seems to increase each time I practise. I feel very much at peace and healed.

After many years of strength training with heavy weights, Qigong has improved my flexibility and rigidness both physically and on an emotional level. I did not realise how rigid and stiff I had become from weight training until I began practising Qigong. It also helped calm anxiety attacks.

I truly believe the practice of Qigong played a huge part in my survival of cancer. The healing aspects of Qigong are underestimated particularly by orthodox medicine. I learnt that I can calm my mind and be still and that I can heal my own body. I believe that Qigong has changed my outlook on life and therefore has attracted like-minded people into my life, something that I have been trying to change for a long time.

When I felt the need to teach Qigong, I searched for a Master and fortunately I was guided to Qigong Master Simon Blow. I commenced with Simon's DVDs and found his instructions and execution of each exercise very easy to follow. I attended several of Simon's workshops and have found him to be very informative, polite and charming. Simon's gentle and calm nature exudes through his workshops and creates a wonderful atmosphere. I am ever so grateful that we have crossed paths along my journey of discovering Qigong. **Angela, Queensland**

I was introduced to Tai Chi in 1987. I had studied acupressure massage in 1977 and still employ this massage technique. When performing certain movements of Tai Chi I immediately felt meridian blockages released and energy pathways connecting.

I was introduced to Qigong in 2000. This powerful exercise routine is impressive and effective. I practise Tai Chi Qigong and medical Qigong exercises regularly and incorporate the principles into everyday activities. My practice of these exercises is usually 1-4 hours per day for 3-5 days per week, but I always use the principles when performing any activity either around the home, work or in the garden.

Qigong is a powerful exercise routine which enhances the body's ability to clear energy blockages and allow our organs to function at maximum efficiency. Qigong stills the mind and activates the body's healing capabilities. Sometimes I feel relaxed, sometimes I feel rejuvenated and sometimes I feel energised, but always I feel peaceful and calm.

Qigong practice is the perfect way to escape from a busy and/or stressful lifestyle. I believe Qigong practice has lessened the onset and intensity of migraines from which I have suffered for many years and has given me a greater appreciation of the power of the body/mind connection.

I have learnt that regular Qigong exercises are an essential part of maintaining a peaceful and healthy mind and body. I have learnt that everyone can benefit from Qigong exercises, from the very young to the very old, from the very sick to the very healthy. Everyone can benefit!

Qigong practice works on many different levels. It provides the practitioner with a greater understanding of their own body and how it works. It allows the mind to relax and let the body move in a co-ordinated and relaxed way, enhancing movement, releasing energy blockages and creating vital synovial fluid into all the joints of our body. I recommend certain Qigong exercises to my clients who all notice a benefit when practising.

Qigong exercise routines vary in time and intensity – if people lack discipline to exercise, Qigong routines provide the perfect balance of exercise and meditation, both essential for optimal body health, along with a healthy and balanced diet.

Body health is not a mystery. All it needs is fresh air, fresh water, balanced diet and exercise. Meditation has also been proven to assist in regenerating the body. If one drinks fresh water, practises Qigong exercises outside in the fresh air and eats a balanced diet, then health will surely follow.

I'm personally training and massaging a gentleman at the moment who has diabetes, high blood pressure and is overweight. His physical appearance 'screams' lung problems to me. He just commenced as a 'fitness' client. I did a basic fitness test on his first session, but in the second session I introduced Shibashi movements 1, 2 and 14 to try and aerate his lungs. His first session with these exercises immediately made a difference to his facial colour. I've known him now for several months and he has always had a 'pasty', unhealthy facial colour. After 20 minutes of Qigong warm up, followed by the Shibashi movements, his face was a beautiful pink colour. His wife even noticed it. Amazing. And ... he loves the movements.
Lee, Victoria

I have been practising Qigong for some twenty years now but have become more serious in the last four years as my understanding of the connection to Traditional Chinese Medicine has grown. I now practise five or six times a week.

Having always been active and interested in maintaining my fitness levels, I found the opportunities for organised activity were limited when I moved to a country area. So when a Tai Chi class was eventually available several years ago I joined up.

Practising Qigong definitely puts a smile on my face. As a practitioner aged 80 years, it is important for me to keep my mobility and brainpower at maximum levels and I feel Qigong can help me to do this if I continue to apply myself (we still have to help ourselves).

An important learning for me has been the acceptance of impermanence and to be thankful for Now. Four years ago my right knee was very painful and it was recommended that I wear a hinged metal brace for support – which certainly relieved the pain – and I was wearing this brace in my Tai Chi classes. However, I was concerned about the restricted use of my leg muscles and took the brace off for increasing periods of time until I no longer used it. My knee still 'creaks' but it is no longer painful and the range of movement is barely restricted. Also my previously elevated blood pressure is coming down since concentrating on the relevant exercises. My kidney function has definitely improved. So for me it all works! An hour of time to follow a routine may seem like a lot but I have found that I achieve far more in the day by starting it off with Qigong exercises and giving myself time to absorb the energy. **Shirley, NSW**

I have been practising Qigong for approximately two years. During winter I do it three times per week but with the days getting longer I can manage five times a week.

I began practising Qigong for health reasons and I was overweight. The doctors could find nothing wrong but I felt as though my body was closing down. I had weight problems all of my life but suddenly decided – no more. Since doing Qigong I have lost 20kg and have done it easily. I'm feeling a lot healthier now, much more flexible. And I'm feeling more in contact with my outer and inner body.

The way I understand Qigong is that the Universe and everything in it is made up of energy. When you do Qigong it's a way to bring this all together and bring balance within.

While I'm doing Qigong I see that it as my time and space. It brings peace inside and makes me feel as though I'm connected to something much bigger than me. It's important to take time to really see oneself. You can give yourself and help everyone around you, but you need time for just yourself. It replenishes your own life force energy. Without that you become ill. You die inside.

I've never had a partner who cared to dance. It doesn't matter anymore – when I do Qigong I dance with the Universe! **Dianne, Victoria**

I have been practising Tai Chi and Qigong for 10 years and I practise every day. It is an extension to my studies in Traditional Chinese Medicine

(TCM) and as a spiritual meditation practice.

My understanding of Qigong is that it is based on the concept of the Dao and TCM and can be used as a health/longevity practice or as a path to enlightenment. Qigong works on both a physical level and an energy level (the two can't be separated). It is designed to balance physiological/psychological/energetic functions of the body and mind and bring us into harmony with universal energy or the Dao.

Qigong helps me to feel physically relaxed and balanced as well as mentally peaceful and calm but energised. It helps with my martial arts training, keeps me calm to deal with the stress of life and helps nourish my kidney yin and jing.

I have become more aware of my conditioning and how this affects my health and how I treat others. I have learned that the more calm and peaceful and balanced I am, the happier I am and the better I treat others and I am clearer about how I speak, think and behave. Through this awareness I have learned that there is a direct relationship between myself and the world around me and that ultimately I am the world I live in – I create it from within. **Bul Hae (Zen Buddhist Monk), Queensland**

Seven years ago I was practising Qigong daily. Now I practise 3-4 times per week. My wife started doing it for dry eyes when I was having trouble with Meniere's disease, for which I was told there was no cure. I started Qigong with good results.

When I practise Qigong I feel peaceful, calm, and centred and I am definitely in better health. I now teach Qigong and notice we get better results outside in the open air than inside. Apart from teaching a clan once a week I also introduce trainee Physical Education teachers to Qigong and meditation. Most of them enjoy it and some use it in their teaching. Last year the final year students asked me to teach them again at their camp each morning (they were introduced to Qigong in 2nd year). I would love to do Qigong more in small groups in nature rather than alone!

Leigh, Victoria
(Senior Lecturer and Program Co-ordinator, Physical Education, RMIT University, School of Medical Sciences, Melbourne, Vic.)

I have been attending weekly Qigong lessons for about five years and try to practise a little each day by incorporating some of the movements into everyday tasks. My main reason for starting Qigong was to increase my mobility and balance.

My knowledge of Qigong is limited but I have read it is an ancient form of gentle exercise originating in China. Although it could be based on martial arts, the movements are very graceful.

I finish each group lesson with a sense of wellbeing, and gain much from the positive energy of other members. Although the group includes people of many ages and types, all are friendly, welcoming and non-competitive. Physically, I feel more confident, more balanced with my walking and generally more mobile.

Spiritually, I am able to find within myself a place of reflection and freedom. Emotionally, I benefit because one concentrates only on the movements, excluding anxious thoughts and worries. Our group is under the guidance of a very encouraging and patient teacher, which generates positive energy. I have learnt to persevere with the practice and welcome the challenge of learning new, complicated movements. I find the benefits of Qigong for me include being able to work within my own capability and making a conscious effort to 'slow down' physically and mentally.
E. Phillips, NSW

I started attending Simon's Qigong classes three years ago. I now practise for about 30 minutes each day. I started going to classes because I read claims on the internet that Qigong could help relieve arthritis pain and that led me to 'give it a go'.

I consider Qigong to be Chinese alchemy. It makes me feel good! Actually, better than good some days! Qigong movements massage and heat my body first thing in the morning. I find the rhythmic breathing very calming and I've avoided lung infections during these past three years. I've also found that a short period of meditation, anywhere, anytime restores lost energy.

Qigong practice has reinforced the idea that I have many elements to my wellbeing and that each one has to operate harmoniously with the others. If they don't, it affects my mind, body and soul.

Simon, your most memorable saying is "go at your own pace…we'll not have exams here…yet." Teaching is a remarkable gift, often not fully appreciated. You are one of those exceptional teachers! And I feel fortunate that I've been one of your students. **Margaret, NSW**

I am doing a life sentence, in the old act, and in early 1994, I started Tai Chi classes with Simon. At first, I too as well as many others, was unsure of the outcome of the course, but with inside pressures and the lack of harmonies, and activities, I found myself thirsting for positive energies. I am now past the initiation class and on my third level with three to go.

Since doing classes, I find myself more positive within my environment here in jail. I can speak warmly and I have more self-confidence to express myself instead of bottling things in. I am able to excel to a depth of achievements not only with Tai Chi but with my sculptures which now have taken on a tradition of years ago.

I must say thanks to Simon and Corrective Services for providing an opportunity of establishing our innerness with the outside world. I personally am astonished with the changes in myself since I started the Tai Chi classes, in fact, watching others around me I can see the energy levels rise within each and every one of them. Once again, thank you.
Name withheld

I've been practicing for about five years and practice six days a week and if time permits sometimes twice a day. I first started reading about some of the amazing healing benefits that Qigong can bring, so I decided to try it for myself.

My understanding initially came from what I had read about Qigong, so as I practise more and more, that understanding becomes more of an experience to be felt as opposed to mere thinking. It constantly amazes me that something that appears so simple can give me such a feeling of wellbeing and inner harmony.

I like to think that I take a certain amount of responsibility for my own health. So I believe the benefits are preventing illness and gaining health and longevity. What I'm learning I believe is an ongoing process. I think Qigong makes me appreciate the present moment more, and that being in the present is all there is.

I find one of the greatest challenges in practicing Qigong is to engage my mind and keep focused on what I'm doing. This is where I believe that the greatest benefits can happen. For me it's not so much the destination but the journey. I am constantly discovering new sensations about myself, both physically and mentally and even sometimes there is a sense of the spiritual where I feel more connected with everything. I feel that my journey is in the early stages and that I have many more years of discovery.
Neville, Victoria

I have been practising Qigong for 10 years and prior to that I was doing Tai Chi for many years. I practise about three times a week but plan to practise daily. The only inhibiter to this has been my farm activities, especially over winter. When I was practising Tai Chi, we also did a little Qigong which I enjoyed.

The total conversion to Qigong happened when I had a car accident and stopped Tai Chi for quite a while and then I started Qigong. Following this I discovered Simon, whom I now look upon as my Qigong Master.

Qigong makes me feel more alive, fit and definitely healthier. Peace of mind always follows and continues through the day and week. Qigong has changed my whole life. I am happier, much more accepting of whatever crops up in life. My body is supple and the benefits are far reaching.

I just love Qigong, but it is also a discipline and this helps to guide my practice. Following Qigong I like to meditate. This gives me a lot of patience with people around and an enormous appetite to enjoy every day of my life. With my love of Qigong and my better lifestyle, I must acknowledge my Master Simon. Perhaps without such a wonderful Master, Qigong may not have had the same results. His patient guidance and warmth has resulted in encouraging and developing my passion. I think Qigong should be introduced to all primary and secondary schools as part of the curriculum. Life is so fast and people have lost the ability to relax and enjoy this beautiful world. Qigong sharpens the senses, calms the mind and enlivens the body, giving the owner of the body a complete sensational feeling of wellbeing. **Virginia, NSW**

CDs – by Simon Blow

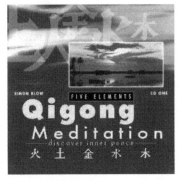

CD1: Five Elements Qigong Meditation

This CD is the perfect introduction to Qigong meditation (Neigong). **Track one** features a 30-minute heart-felt guided meditation to help bring love and light from the universe into your body. It harmonises the Five Elements – Fire, Earth, Metal, Water and Wood – with the corresponding organs of the body, respectively the heart, spleen, lungs, kidney and liver. This is one of the foundations of Chinese Qigong. Let Qigong Master Simon Blow help harmonise the elements of the universe with the energy of your body by using colour and positive images. **Track two** provides 30 minutes of relaxing music by inspiring composer Dale Nougher.

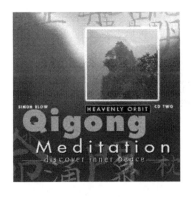

CD2: Heavenly Orbit Qigong Meditation

This CD is intended for the intermediate student. **Track one** takes you through a 30-minute guided meditation using your awareness to stimulate the energy centres around the body and open all the meridians. The circulation of Qi (Chi) around the Heavenly Orbit is one of the foundations of Chinese Qigong. The energy rising up the back 'Du' channel harmonises with the energy descending down the front 'Ren' channel, helping balance the energy of the body. Master Simon Blow guides you to open the energy centres of your own body to create harmony with the universe. **Track two** provides 30 minutes of relaxing music by Dale Nougher.

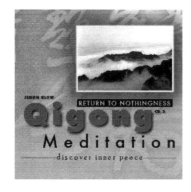

CD3: Return to Nothingness Qigong Meditation

This CD is intended for the advanced student and those wanting a healing night-practice. One of the aims of Qigong is to allow our internal energy (Qi) to harmonise with the external energy (Qi) allowing our consciousness to merge with the universe. When we enter into a deep sleep or meditation all the meridians start to open and much healing can take place. In this 20-minute guided meditation Simon Blow assists you in guiding your energy through your body and harmonising with the energy of the universe. Track two provides 30 minutes of healing music by Dale Nougher.

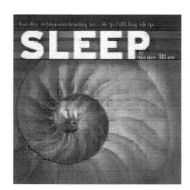

Sleep

Sleep is necessary to maintain life, alongside breathing, eating, drinking, and exercising of the mind and body. Without a good six to eight hours of sleep each night it can be hard to live a quality, balanced, fulfilling life. When we sleep it's a time to rest and rejuvenate the mind and body and to release the physical, mental and emotional stress that has built up during the day. This also helps uplift us spiritually.

It's a time to rest; it's time for a good night's sleep. Let Simon Blow's soothing voice, along with Dale Nougher's beautiful piano music and the natural sounds of the ocean, help guide you to release the tension of the day and enable you to enter a deep, fulfilling sleep.

Book/DVD sets – by Simon Blow

"About 18 months ago I started to practise Qigong as I knew that it would improve my health. I needed to do it regularly, ideally every day, but being in a rural area presented logistical problems. I discovered Simon's DVD and commenced daily practice. The great advantage for me was that I didn't have to travel to classes and could do them whenever I felt like it. Since that time I have noticed great improvement in my overall wellbeing. It has helped me to reinvent my clinical practice as a holistic massage practitioner. A number of my clients now have Simon's DVD and I feel this is helping them to both improve their health and well being, and to empower themselves." **Robin Godson-King (Holistic Massage Practitioner)**

(Each set contains a DVD plus a book that provides diagrams and instructions for the movements contained on the DVD. The book also includes interesting reading about the practice of Qigong as well as inspirational stories.)

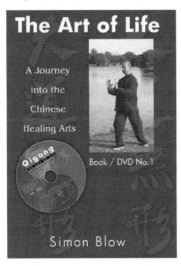

The Art of Life

'The Art of Life' presents the Qigong styles that were taught to me in Australia: the Taiji Qigong Shibashi, which I learned as an instructor with the Australian Academy of Tai Chi from 1990 to 1995; and the Ba Duan Jin standing form, commonly known as the Eight Pieces of Brocade, taught to me in 1996 by Sifu John Dolic in Sydney.

This is the perfect introduction to this ancient art and is suitable for new and continuing students of all ages. The book follows the DVD and contains three sections: **1. Warm up** – gentle movements loosen all the major joints of the body, lubricating the tendons and helping increase blood and energy circulation. It is beneficial for most arthritic conditions; **2. Ba Duan Jin or Eight Pieces of Brocade** – this is the best known and most widely practised form of Qigong throughout the world, also known as Daoist Yoga. The movements stretch all the major muscles, massage organs and open the meridians of the body; **3. Taiji Qigong Shibashi** – this popular practice is made up of eighteen flowing movements. The gentle movements harmonise the mind, body and breath. Total running time: 55 minutes.

"Tai Chi Qigong is a gentle way of exercising the whole body and provides long-term benefits. I recommend it to my patients as an effective way of improving muscle tone and joint mobility. Those who practise regularly have fewer problems with their muscles and joints and often report an increased sense of health and wellbeing. This is an excellent video with clear and simple instruction."
Roman Maslak. B.A. (Hons), D.O. Osteopath

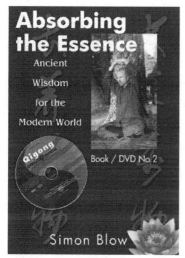

Absorbing the Essence

'Absorbing the Essence' comprises the Qigong cultivation techniques that were taught to me by Grand Master Zhong Yunlong in 1999 and 2000 at Wudangshan or Wudang Mountain. Wudang is one of the sacred Daoist Mountains of China and is renowned for the development of Taiji.

This DVD and book is for the intermediate student and for people with experience in meditation. It contains three sections: **1. Warm up** – the same as in The Art of Life DVD; **2. Wudang Longevity Qigong** – this sequence of gentle, flowing movements stimulates the Heavenly Orbit, absorbing the primordial energy from the environment and letting the negativity dissolve into the distance; **3. Sitting Ba Duan Jin** – this 30-minute sequence includes eight sections with exercises to stimulate different organs and meridians of the body. It is practised in a seated position on a chair or cushion – ideal for people who have discomfort whilst standing. These practices originated from the famous Purple Cloud Monastery at the sacred Wudang Mountain in China. Total running time: 60 minutes.

"Simon Blow of Australia has twice travelled (1999, 2000) to Mt Wudang Shan Daoist Wushu College to learn Taiji Hunyuan Zhuang (Longevity) Qigong and Badajin Nurturing Life Qigong and through his study has absorbed the essence of these teachings. Therefore, I specially grant Simon the authority to teach these, spreading the knowledge of these Qigong methods he has learnt at Mt Wudang to contribute to the wellbeing of the human race. May the Meritorious Deeds Be Infinite."
Grand Master Zhong Yunlong, Daoist Priest and Director,
Mt Wudang Shan Taoist Wushu College, China, September 24, 2000.

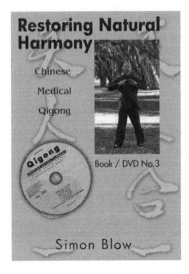

Restoring Natural Harmony

This DVD and book is for the advanced student or for the person wanting to learn specific Traditional Chinese Medicine self-healing exercises. Each section works on a different organ meridian system of the body – Spleen, Lungs, Kidney, Liver and Heart – which relate to the Five Elements – Earth, Metal, Water, Wood and Fire. Guigen Qigong originated from Dr Xu Hongtao, a Qigong Specialist Doctor from the Xiyuan Hospital in Beijing. These internal exercises help regulate the meridian system bringing harmony to mind, body and spirit. Total running time: 75 minutes.

"Simon Blow first visited our hospital in 2002. I was impressed with his knowledge and commitment to Qigong. He returned in 2004 to study Chinese Medical Qigong. Simon is a gifted teacher: he has the rare ability to inspire others and impart to them the healing benefits of Qigong."
Dr Xu Hongtao, Qigong and Tuina Department, Xiyuan Hospital Beijing, China.

"This DVD – the third by the impressively qualified Sydney-based Simon Blow – serves two purposes. Firstly, it is so attractively produced that the curious would surely be induced to investigate further. Secondly, for those already practising, it provides a mnemonic device much more useful than a series of still pictures." **Review by Adyar Bookshop, Sydney 2005.**

These are not medical devices and should not be used to replace any existing medical treatment. Always consult with your health provider if uncertain.

To order products or for more information on:
- Regular classes in Sydney for new and continuing students
- Workshops or if you would be interested in helping organise a workshop in your local area
- Residential Qigong and Meditation retreats
- China Qigong Study Tours for students and advanced training
- Talks, corporate classes, training and presentations
- Wholesale enquiries

Please contact:

Simon Blow
PO Box 446
Summer Hill, NSW 2130
Sydney Australia

Ph: +61 (0)2 9559 8153

Web: **www.simonblowqigong.com**

CDs and Book/DVDs can be ordered online and shipped nationally and internationally.

Bibliography

Publications

Blow, Simon. *Survey of Benefits of Qigong Practice with a Drug Rehabilitation Population*, presented at the World Medical Qigong Conference, Beijing 2004.

Wu Changguo. *Basic Theory of Traditional Chinese Medicine*. China: Publishing House of Shanghai University of Traditional Chinese Medicine, 2002.

Ni Hua-Ching. Tao: *The Subtle Universal Law and the Integral Way of Life* (2nd edn). California: Seven Star Communications Group, Inc., 1995.

Ni Hua-Ching. *Esoteric Tao Teh Ching*. California: Seven Star Communications Group, Inc., 1992.

Liu Qingshan. *Chinese Fitness*. Massachusetts: YMAA Publication Centre, 1997.

Sancier, K.M., Holman, D. Multifaceted Health Benefits of Medical Qigong, *J. Alt Compl Med.* 10(1):163-166, 2004.

Websites

ABC News-Health:
http://abcnews.go.com/Health/Story?id=5287805&page=1

Meditation Research: **www.researchingmeditation.org**

Meditation Research Institute: **www.meditationresearchinstitute.org/**

National Centre for Complementary and Alternative Medicine: **http://nccam.nih.gov/health/meditation/overview.htm**

Psychology Today: **www.psychologytoday.com/articles/200105/the-science-meditation**

Qigong Institute: **www.qigonginstitute.org**

Meridian Diagrams

Original meridian diagrams sourced from:
Wu Changguo. *Basic Theory of Traditional Chinese Medicine*. China: Publishing House of Shanghai University of Traditional Chinese Medicine.

Made in the USA
San Bernardino, CA
22 January 2018